FREE Study Skills DVD Offer

Dear Customer,

Thank you for your purchase from Mometrix! We consider it an honor and a privilege that you have purchased our product and we want to ensure your satisfaction.

As a way of showing our appreciation and to help us better serve you, we have developed a Study Skills DVD that we would like to give you for <u>FREE</u>. This DVD covers our *best practices* for getting ready for your exam, from how to use our study materials to how to best prepare for the day of the test.

All that we ask is that you email us with feedback that would describe your experience so far with our product. Good, bad, or indifferent, we want to know what you think!

To get your FREE Study Skills DVD, email freedvd@mometrix.com with *FREE STUDY SKILLS DVD* in the subject line and the following information in the body of the email:

- The name of the product you purchased.
- Your product rating on a scale of 1-5, with 5 being the highest rating.
- Your feedback. It can be long, short, or anything in between. We just want to know your impressions and experience so far with our product. (Good feedback might include how our study material met your needs and ways we might be able to make it even better. You could highlight features that you found helpful or features that you think we should add.)
- Your full name and shipping address where you would like us to send your free DVD.

If you have any questions or concerns, please don't hesitate to contact me directly.

Thanks again!

Sincerely,

Jay Willis
Vice President
jay.willis@mometrix.com
1-800-673-8175

EMT
Exam Study Guide
2019 & 2020

SECRETS

Study Guide
Your Key to Exam Success

EMT Basic Exam Prep Secrets &
Practice Test Questions for the
NREMT Emergency Medical
Technician Exam (Updated for the
Current EMT Cognitive Exam Test Plan)

Dear Future Exam Success Story:

First of all, **THANK YOU** for purchasing Mometrix study materials!

Second, congratulations! You are one of the few determined test-takers who are committed to doing whatever it takes to excel on your exam. **You have come to the right place.** We developed these study materials with one goal in mind: to deliver you the information you need in a format that's concise and easy to use.

In addition to optimizing your guide for the content of the test, we've outlined our recommended steps for breaking down the preparation process into small, attainable goals so you can make sure you stay on track.

We've also analyzed the entire test-taking process, identifying the most common pitfalls and showing how you can overcome them and be ready for any curveball the test throws you.

Standardized testing is one of the biggest obstacles on your road to success, which only increases the importance of doing well in the high-pressure, high-stakes environment of test day. Your results on this test could have a significant impact on your future, and this guide provides the information and practical advice to help you achieve your full potential on test day.

Your success is our success

We would love to hear from you! If you would like to share the story of your exam success or if you have any questions or comments in regard to our products, please contact us at **800-673-8175** or **support@mometrix.com**.

Thanks again for your business and we wish you continued success!

Sincerely,
The Mometrix Test Preparation Team

Need more help? Check out our flashcards at: http://MometrixFlashcards.com/EMT

TABLE OF CONTENTS

Introduction

Thank you for purchasing this resource! You have made the choice to prepare yourself for a test that could have a huge impact on your future, and this guide is designed to help you be fully ready for test day. Obviously, it's important to have a solid understanding of the test material, but you also need to be prepared for the unique environment and stressors of the test, so that you can perform to the best of your abilities.

For this purpose, the first section that appears in this guide is the **Secret Keys**. We've devoted countless hours to meticulously researching what works and what doesn't, and we've boiled down our findings to the five most impactful steps you can take to improve your performance on the test. We start at the beginning with study planning and move through the preparation process, all the way to the testing strategies that will help you get the most out of what you know when you're finally sitting in front of the test.

We recommend that you start preparing for your test as far in advance as possible. However, if you've bought this guide as a last-minute study resource and only have a few days before your test, we recommend that you skip over the first two Secret Keys since they address a long-term study plan.

If you struggle with **test anxiety**, we strongly encourage you to check out our recommendations for how you can overcome it. Test anxiety is a formidable foe, but it can be beaten, and we want to make sure you have the tools you need to defeat it.

Secret Key #1 – Plan Big, Study Small

There's a lot riding on your performance. If you want to ace this test, you're going to need to keep your skills sharp and the material fresh in your mind. You need a plan that lets you review everything you need to know while still fitting in your schedule. We'll break this strategy down into three categories.

Information Organization

Start with the information you already have: the official test outline. From this, you can make a complete list of all the concepts you need to cover before the test. Organize these concepts into groups that can be studied together, and create a list of any related vocabulary you need to learn so you can brush up on any difficult terms. You'll want to keep this vocabulary list handy once you actually start studying since you may need to add to it along the way.

Time Management

Once you have your set of study concepts, decide how to spread them out over the time you have left before the test. Break your study plan into small, clear goals so you have a manageable task for each day and know exactly what you're doing. Then just focus on one small step at a time. When you manage your time this way, you don't need to spend hours at a time studying. Studying a small block of content for a short period each day helps you retain information better and avoid stressing over how much you have left to do. You can relax knowing that you have a plan to cover everything in time. In order for this strategy to be effective though, you have to start studying early and stick to your schedule. Avoid the exhaustion and futility that comes from last-minute cramming!

Study Environment

The environment you study in has a big impact on your learning. Studying in a coffee shop, while probably more enjoyable, is not likely to be as fruitful as studying in a quiet room. It's important to keep distractions to a minimum. You're only planning to study for a short block of time, so make the most of it. Don't pause to check your phone or get up to find a snack. It's also important to **avoid multitasking**. Research has consistently shown that multitasking will make your studying dramatically less effective. Your study area should also be comfortable and well-lit so you don't have the distraction of straining your eyes or sitting on an uncomfortable chair.

The time of day you study is also important. You want to be rested and alert. Don't wait until just before bedtime. Study when you'll be most likely to comprehend and remember. Even better, if you know what time of day your test will be, set that time aside for study. That way your brain will be used to working on that subject at that specific time and you'll have a better chance of recalling information.

Finally, it can be helpful to team up with others who are studying for the same test. Your actual studying should be done in as isolated an environment as possible, but the work of organizing the information and setting up the study plan can be divided up. In between study sessions, you can discuss with your teammates the concepts that you're all studying and quiz each other on the details. Just be sure that your teammates are as serious about the test as you are. If you find that your study time is being replaced with social time, you might need to find a new team.

Secret Key #2 – Make Your Studying Count

You're devoting a lot of time and effort to preparing for this test, so you want to be absolutely certain it will pay off. This means doing more than just reading the content and hoping you can remember it on test day. It's important to make every minute of study count. There are two main areas you can focus on to make your studying count:

Retention

It doesn't matter how much time you study if you can't remember the material. You need to make sure you are retaining the concepts. To check your retention of the information you're learning, try recalling it at later times with minimal prompting. Try carrying around flashcards and glance at one or two from time to time or ask a friend who's also studying for the test to quiz you.

To enhance your retention, look for ways to put the information into practice so that you can apply it rather than simply recalling it. If you're using the information in practical ways, it will be much easier to remember. Similarly, it helps to solidify a concept in your mind if you're not only reading it to yourself but also explaining it to someone else. Ask a friend to let you teach them about a concept you're a little shaky on (or speak aloud to an imaginary audience if necessary). As you try to summarize, define, give examples, and answer your friend's questions, you'll understand the concepts better and they will stay with you longer. Finally, step back for a big picture view and ask yourself how each piece of information fits with the whole subject. When you link the different concepts together and see them working together as a whole, it's easier to remember the individual components.

Finally, practice showing your work on any multi-step problems, even if you're just studying. Writing out each step you take to solve a problem will help solidify the process in your mind, and you'll be more likely to remember it during the test.

Modality

Modality simply refers to the means or method by which you study. Choosing a study modality that fits your own individual learning style is crucial. No two people learn best in exactly the same way, so it's important to know your strengths and use them to your advantage.

For example, if you learn best by visualization, focus on visualizing a concept in your mind and draw an image or a diagram. Try color-coding your notes, illustrating them, or creating symbols that will trigger your mind to recall a learned concept. If you learn best by hearing or discussing information, find a study partner who learns the same way or read aloud to yourself. Think about how to put the information in your own words. Imagine that you are giving a lecture on the topic and record yourself so you can listen to it later.

For any learning style, flashcards can be helpful. Organize the information so you can take advantage of spare moments to review. Underline key words or phrases. Use different colors for different categories. Mnemonic devices (such as creating a short list in which every item starts with the same letter) can also help with retention. Find what works best for you and use it to store the information in your mind most effectively and easily.

Secret Key #3 – Practice the Right Way

Your success on test day depends not only on how many hours you put into preparing, but also on whether you prepared the right way. It's good to check along the way to see if your studying is paying off. One of the most effective ways to do this is by taking practice tests to evaluate your progress. Practice tests are useful because they show exactly where you need to improve. Every time you take a practice test, pay special attention to these three groups of questions:

- The questions you got wrong
- The questions you had to guess on, even if you guessed right
- The questions you found difficult or slow to work through

This will show you exactly what your weak areas are, and where you need to devote more study time. Ask yourself why each of these questions gave you trouble. Was it because you didn't understand the material? Was it because you didn't remember the vocabulary? Do you need more repetitions on this type of question to build speed and confidence? Dig into those questions and figure out how you can strengthen your weak areas as you go back to review the material.

Additionally, many practice tests have a section explaining the answer choices. It can be tempting to read the explanation and think that you now have a good understanding of the concept. However, an explanation likely only covers part of the question's broader context. Even if the explanation makes sense, **go back and investigate** every concept related to the question until you're positive you have a thorough understanding.

As you go along, keep in mind that the practice test is just that: practice. Memorizing these questions and answers will not be very helpful on the actual test because it is unlikely to have any of the same exact questions. If you only know the right answers to the sample questions, you won't be prepared for the real thing. **Study the concepts** until you understand them fully, and then you'll be able to answer any question that shows up on the test.

It's important to wait on the practice tests until you're ready. If you take a test on your first day of study, you may be overwhelmed by the amount of material covered and how much you need to learn. Work up to it gradually.

On test day, you'll need to be prepared for answering questions, managing your time, and using the test-taking strategies you've learned. It's a lot to balance, like a mental marathon that will have a big impact on your future. Like training for a marathon, you'll need to start slowly and work your way up. When test day arrives, you'll be ready.

Start with the strategies you've read in the first two Secret Keys—plan your course and study in the way that works best for you. If you have time, consider using multiple study resources to get different approaches to the same concepts. It can be helpful to see difficult concepts from more than one angle. Then find a good source for practice tests. Many times, the test website will suggest potential study resources or provide sample tests.

Practice Test Strategy

If you're able to find at least three practice tests, we recommend this strategy:

1. Take the first test with no time constraints and with your notes and study guide handy. Take your time and focus on applying the strategies you've learned.
2. Take the second practice test open-book as well, but set a timer and practice pacing yourself to finish in time.
3. Take any other practice tests as if it were test day. Set a timer and put away your study materials. Sit at a table or desk in a quiet room, imagine yourself at the testing center, and answer questions as quickly and accurately as possible.
4. Keep repeating step 3 on a regular basis until you run out of practice tests or it's time for the actual test. Your mind will be ready for the schedule and stress of test day, and you'll be able to focus on recalling the material you've learned.

Secret Key #4 – Pace Yourself

Once you're fully prepared for the material on the test, your biggest challenge on test day will be managing your time. Just knowing that the clock is ticking can make you panic even if you have plenty of time left. Work on pacing yourself so you can build confidence against the time constraints of the exam. Pacing is a difficult skill to master, especially in a high-pressure environment, so **practice is vital**.

Set time expectations for your pace based on how much time is available. For example, if a section has 60 questions and the time limit is 30 minutes, you know you have to average 30 seconds or less per question in order to answer them all. Although 30 seconds is the hard limit, set 25 seconds per question as your goal, so you reserve extra time to spend on harder questions. When you budget extra time for the harder questions, you no longer have any reason to stress when those questions take longer to answer.

Don't let this time expectation distract you from working through the test at a calm, steady pace, but keep it in mind so you don't spend too much time on any one question. Recognize that taking extra time on one question you don't understand may keep you from answering two that you do understand later in the test. If your time limit for a question is up and you're still not sure of the answer, mark it and move on, and come back to it later if the time and the test format allow. If the testing format doesn't allow you to return to earlier questions, just make an educated guess; then put it out of your mind and move on.

On the easier questions, be careful not to rush. It may seem wise to hurry through them so you have more time for the challenging ones, but it's not worth missing one if you know the concept and just didn't take the time to read the question fully. Work efficiently but make sure you understand the question and have looked at all of the answer choices, since more than one may seem right at first.

Even if you're paying attention to the time, you may find yourself a little behind at some point. You should speed up to get back on track, but do so wisely. Don't panic; just take a few seconds less on each question until you're caught up. Don't guess without thinking, but do look through the answer choices and eliminate any you know are wrong. If you can get down to two choices, it is often worthwhile to guess from those. Once you've chosen an answer, move on and don't dwell on any that you skipped or had to hurry through. If a question was taking too long, chances are it was one of the harder ones, so you weren't as likely to get it right anyway.

On the other hand, if you find yourself getting ahead of schedule, it may be beneficial to slow down a little. The more quickly you work, the more likely you are to make a careless mistake that will affect your score. You've budgeted time for each question, so don't be afraid to spend that time. Practice an efficient but careful pace to get the most out of the time you have.

Secret Key #5 – Have a Plan for Guessing

When you're taking the test, you may find yourself stuck on a question. Some of the answer choices seem better than others, but you don't see the one answer choice that is obviously correct. What do you do?

The scenario described above is very common, yet most test takers have not effectively prepared for it. Developing and practicing a plan for guessing may be one of the single most effective uses of your time as you get ready for the exam.

In developing your plan for guessing, there are three questions to address:

- When should you start the guessing process?
- How should you narrow down the choices?
- Which answer should you choose?

When to Start the Guessing Process

Unless your plan for guessing is to select C every time (which, despite its merits, is not what we recommend), you need to leave yourself enough time to apply your answer elimination strategies. Since you have a limited amount of time for each question, that means that if you're going to give yourself the best shot at guessing correctly, you have to decide quickly whether or not you will guess.

Of course, the best-case scenario is that you don't have to guess at all, so first, see if you can answer the question based on your knowledge of the subject and basic reasoning skills. Focus on the key words in the question and try to jog your memory of related topics. Give yourself a chance to bring the knowledge to mind, but once you realize that you don't have (or you can't access) the knowledge you need to answer the question, it's time to start the guessing process.

It's almost always better to start the guessing process too early than too late. It only takes a few seconds to remember something and answer the question from knowledge. Carefully eliminating wrong answer choices takes longer. Plus, going through the process of eliminating answer choices can actually help jog your memory.

Summary: Start the guessing process as soon as you decide that you can't answer the question based on your knowledge.

How to Narrow Down the Choices

The next chapter in this book (**Test-Taking Strategies**) includes a wide range of strategies for how to approach questions and how to look for answer choices to eliminate. You will definitely want to read those carefully, practice them, and figure out which ones work best for you. Here though, we're going to address a mindset rather than a particular strategy.

Your chances of guessing an answer correctly depend on how many options you are choosing from.

How many choices you have	How likely you are to guess correctly
5	20%
4	25%
3	33%
2	50%
1	100%

You can see from this chart just how valuable it is to be able to eliminate incorrect answers and make an educated guess, but there are two things that many test takers do that cause them to miss out on the benefits of guessing:

- Accidentally eliminating the correct answer
- Selecting an answer based on an impression

We'll look at the first one here, and the second one in the next section.

To avoid accidentally eliminating the correct answer, we recommend a thought exercise called **the $5 challenge**. In this challenge, you only eliminate an answer choice from contention if you are willing to bet $5 on it being wrong. Why $5? Five dollars is a small but not insignificant amount of money. It's an amount you could afford to lose but wouldn't want to throw away. And while losing $5 once might not hurt too much, doing it twenty times will set you back $100. In the same way, each small decision you make—eliminating a choice here, guessing on a question there—won't by itself impact your score very much, but when you put them all together, they can make a big difference. By holding each answer choice elimination decision to a higher standard, you can reduce the risk of accidentally eliminating the correct answer.

The $5 challenge can also be applied in a positive sense: If you are willing to bet $5 that an answer choice *is* correct, go ahead and mark it as correct.

Summary: Only eliminate an answer choice if you are willing to bet $5 that it is wrong.

Which Answer to Choose

You're taking the test. You've run into a hard question and decided you'll have to guess. You've eliminated all the answer choices you're willing to bet $5 on. Now you have to pick an answer. Why do we even need to talk about this? Why can't you just pick whichever one you feel like when the time comes?

The answer to these questions is that if you don't come into the test with a plan, you'll rely on your impression to select an answer choice, and if you do that, you risk falling into a trap. The test writers know that everyone who takes their test will be guessing on some of the questions, so they intentionally write wrong answer choices to seem plausible. You still have to pick an answer though, and if the wrong answer choices are designed to look right, how can you ever be sure that you're not falling for their trap? The best solution we've found to this dilemma is to take the decision out of your hands entirely. Here is the process we recommend:

Once you've eliminated any choices that you are confident (willing to bet $5) are wrong, select the first remaining choice as your answer.

Whether you choose to select the first remaining choice, the second, or the last, the important thing is that you use some preselected standard. Using this approach guarantees that you will not be enticed into selecting an answer choice that looks right, because you are not basing your decision on how the answer choices look.

This is not meant to make you question your knowledge. Instead, it is to help you recognize the difference between your knowledge and your impressions. There's a huge difference between thinking an answer is right because of what you know, and thinking an answer is right because it looks or sounds like it should be right.

Summary: To ensure that your selection is appropriately random, make a predetermined selection from among all answer choices you have not eliminated.

Test-Taking Strategies

This section contains a list of test-taking strategies that you may find helpful as you work through the test. By taking what you know and applying logical thought, you can maximize your chances of answering any question correctly!

It is very important to realize that every question is different and every person is different: no single strategy will work on every question, and no single strategy will work for every person. That's why we've included all of them here, so you can try them out and determine which ones work best for different types of questions and which ones work best for you.

Question Strategies

Read Carefully

Read the question and answer choices carefully. Don't miss the question because you misread the terms. You have plenty of time to read each question thoroughly and make sure you understand what is being asked. Yet a happy medium must be attained, so don't waste too much time. You must read carefully, but efficiently.

Contextual Clues

Look for contextual clues. If the question includes a word you are not familiar with, look at the immediate context for some indication of what the word might mean. Contextual clues can often give you all the information you need to decipher the meaning of an unfamiliar word. Even if you can't determine the meaning, you may be able to narrow down the possibilities enough to make a solid guess at the answer to the question.

Prefixes

If you're having trouble with a word in the question or answer choices, try dissecting it. Take advantage of every clue that the word might include. Prefixes and suffixes can be a huge help. Usually they allow you to determine a basic meaning. Pre- means before, post- means after, pro - is positive, de- is negative. From prefixes and suffixes, you can get an idea of the general meaning of the word and try to put it into context.

Hedge Words

Watch out for critical hedge words, such as *likely, may, can, sometimes, often, almost, mostly, usually, generally, rarely*, and *sometimes*. Question writers insert these hedge phrases to cover every possibility. Often an answer choice will be wrong simply because it leaves no room for exception. Be on guard for answer choices that have definitive words such as *exactly* and *always*.

Switchback Words

Stay alert for *switchbacks*. These are the words and phrases frequently used to alert you to shifts in thought. The most common switchback words are *but, although,* and *however*. Others include *nevertheless, on the other hand, even though, while, in spite of, despite, regardless of*. Switchback words are important to catch because they can change the direction of the question or an answer choice.

- 10 -

Face Value

When in doubt, use common sense. Accept the situation in the problem at face value. Don't read too much into it. These problems will not require you to make wild assumptions. If you have to go beyond creativity and warp time or space in order to have an answer choice fit the question, then you should move on and consider the other answer choices. These are normal problems rooted in reality. The applicable relationship or explanation may not be readily apparent, but it is there for you to figure out. Use your common sense to interpret anything that isn't clear.

Answer Choice Strategies

Answer Selection

The most thorough way to pick an answer choice is to identify and eliminate wrong answers until only one is left, then confirm it is the correct answer. Sometimes an answer choice may immediately seem right, but be careful. The test writers will usually put more than one reasonable answer choice on each question, so take a second to read all of them and make sure that the other choices are not equally obvious. As long as you have time left, it is better to read every answer choice than to pick the first one that looks right without checking the others.

Eliminate Answers

Eliminate answer choices as soon as you realize they are wrong, but make sure you consider all possibilities. If you are eliminating answer choices and realize that the last one you are left with is also wrong, don't panic. Start over and consider each choice again. There may be something you missed the first time that you will realize on the second pass.

Avoid Fact Traps

Don't be distracted by an answer choice that is factually true but doesn't answer the question. You are looking for the choice that answers the question. Stay focused on what the question is asking for so you don't accidentally pick an answer that is true but incorrect. Always go back to the question and make sure the answer choice you've selected actually answers the question and is not merely a true statement.

Extreme Statements

In general, you should avoid answers that put forth extreme actions as standard practice or proclaim controversial ideas as established fact. An answer choice that states the "process should be used in certain situations, if..." is much more likely to be correct than one that states the "process should be discontinued completely." The first is a calm rational statement and doesn't even make a definitive, uncompromising stance, using a hedge word *if* to provide wiggle room, whereas the second choice is a radical idea and far more extreme.

Benchmark

As you read through the answer choices and you come across one that seems to answer the question well, mentally select that answer choice. This is not your final answer, but it's the one that will help you evaluate the other answer choices. The one that you selected is your benchmark or standard for judging each of the other answer choices. Every other answer choice must be compared to your benchmark. That choice is correct until proven otherwise by another answer choice beating it. If you find a better answer, then that one becomes your new benchmark. Once you've decided that no other choice answers the question as well as your benchmark, you have your final answer.

Predict the Answer

Before you even start looking at the answer choices, it is often best to try to predict the answer. When you come up with the answer on your own, it is easier to avoid distractions and traps because you will know exactly what to look for. The right answer choice is unlikely to be word-for-word what you came up with, but it should be a close match. Even if you are confident that you have the right answer, you should still take the time to read each option before moving on.

General Strategies

Tough Questions

If you are stumped on a problem or it appears too hard or too difficult, don't waste time. Move on! Remember though, if you can quickly check for obviously incorrect answer choices, your chances of guessing correctly are greatly improved. Before you completely give up, at least try to knock out a couple of possible answers. Eliminate what you can and then guess at the remaining answer choices before moving on.

Check Your Work

Since you will probably not know every term listed and the answer to every question, it is important that you get credit for the ones that you do know. Don't miss any questions through careless mistakes. If at all possible, try to take a second to look back over your answer selection and make sure you've selected the correct answer choice and haven't made a costly careless mistake (such as marking an answer choice that you didn't mean to mark). This quick double check should more than pay for itself in caught mistakes for the time it costs.

Pace Yourself

It's easy to be overwhelmed when you're looking at a page full of questions; your mind is confused and full of random thoughts, and the clock is ticking down faster than you would like. Calm down and maintain the pace that you have set for yourself. Especially as you get down to the last few minutes of the test, don't let the small numbers on the clock make you panic. As long as you are on track by monitoring your pace, you are guaranteed to have time for each question.

Don't Rush

It is very easy to make errors when you are in a hurry. Maintaining a fast pace in answering questions is pointless if it makes you miss questions that you would have gotten right otherwise. Test writers like to include distracting information and wrong answers that seem right. Taking a little extra time to avoid careless mistakes can make all the difference in your test score. Find a pace that allows you to be confident in the answers that you select.

Keep Moving

Panicking will not help you pass the test, so do your best to stay calm and keep moving. Taking deep breaths and going through the answer elimination steps you practiced can help to break through a stress barrier and keep your pace.

Final Notes

The combination of a solid foundation of content knowledge and the confidence that comes from practicing your plan for applying that knowledge is the key to maximizing your performance on test day. As your foundation of content knowledge is built up and strengthened, you'll find that the strategies included in this chapter become more and more effective in helping you quickly sift through the distractions and traps of the test to isolate the correct answer.

Now it's time to move on to the test content chapters of this book, but be sure to keep your goal in mind. As you read, think about how you will be able to apply this information on the test. If you've already seen sample questions for the test and you have an idea of the question format and style, try to come up with questions of your own that you can answer based on what you're reading. This will give you valuable practice applying your knowledge in the same ways you can expect to on test day.

Good luck and good studying!

Preparatory

EMS Systems

The National Highway Traffic Safety Administration (NHTSA) is the lead agency for coordinating and promoting evidence-based emergency medical services (EMS) (fire based, third service, and hospital based) and the 9-1-1 system. The public safety answering point (PSAP) is the designated call-receiving site that directs calls to the appropriate emergency services. Each state defines the scope of practice, licensure, and credentialing for prehospital personnel and sets education standards based on national EMS standards. The advanced emergency medical technician (AEMT) is expected to maintain certification through maintenance of skills and continuing education and should exhibit professional behavior, including working with integrity and empathy, being an effective member of a team, showing respect and tact, maintaining a professional appearance, communicating effectively, and advocating for patients. The AEMT must be alert to patient safety and recognize that most errors result from skills-based, rules-based, and knowledge-based failures. Error reduction requires the use of decision aids and protocols, asking for assistance when appropriate, questioning assumptions, and debriefing calls.

Patient Safety and High-Risk Situations

Up to 98,000 patients die each year because of medical errors. Patients are especially at risk of further injury or death in high-risk situations and activities such as the following:

- Hand-off: A standard procedure, such as SBAR, should be used, as follows:
    - (S) = Situation: Overview of current situation and important issues.
    - (B) = Background: Important history and issues leading to current situation.
    - (A) = Assessment: Summary of important facts and condition.
    - (R) = Recommendation: Actions needed.

- Communications: Problems may result in delayed or inadequate care, wrong address, or wrong destination.
- Dropping: Patients can be easily dropped if the gurney isn't positioned properly or if too few personnel are involved in transport.
- Ambulance crashes: Unnecessary speeding and failing to stop at intersections are the most common causes of ambulance crashes.
- Inadequate spinal immobilization: If unsure, it's always best to immobilize.
- Medication errors: Administration of wrong medication, wrong mode of administration, and wrong dosage.

Roles and Responsibilities of EMS Personnel

Roles and responsibilities of EMS personnel include the following:

- Maintain the readiness of all equipment, including disinfecting, packaging, and storing.
- Monitor personal safety, patient safety, and the safety of others on the scene.
- Evaluate the scene for additional resources when indicated.
- Gain access to the patient only when it is safe to do so.
- Perform an assessment of the patient's condition and needs.
- Provide emergency medical care as needed (or until additional resources arrive).
- Provide emotional support to the patient, family, and other providers.

- Maintain the continuity of care.
- Ensure that medical and legal standards are upheld and that patient privacy is protected.
- Communicate with others and maintain community relations.
- Practice professional behavior (integrity, self-motivation, self-confidence, tact, respect, and professional appearance).
- Maintain certification and meet continuing education requirements.

National EMS Education Agenda for the Future: A Systems Approach

The **National EMS Education Agenda for the Future: A Systems Approach** proposed an education system for EMS with five primary components, establishing the following goals for 2010 and 2020:

1. Core content: Core content to be developed by the EMS medical community, educators, and providers under leadership of the National Highway Traffic Safety Administration (NHTSA) to ensure consistency of content and reciprocity of certification. The core content should be tied to licensure and accreditation.
2. Scope-of-practice model: National models to be used by states for all levels of EMS certification/licensure.
3. Education standards: Standards that are developed by EMS educators with input from the medical community and regulators and that are peer reviewed.
4. Education program accreditation: A single national accreditation agency will develop standards and guidelines.
5. EMS certification: Four levels of national certification with different educational requirements, standards, scopes of practice, and certification: (1) entry-level emergency medical responder (EMR), (2) next-level emergency medical technician (EMT), (3) advanced EMT (AEMT), and (4) paramedic.

Quality Improvement

Quality improvement requires that an organization or system continually evaluates processes and outcomes and takes measures to improve the quality of care. The focus of quality improvement is on patient safety in access, provision of care, transport, and hand-off. Errors are often related to these different types of failures:

- Skills-based: Includes slips and mistakes. Slips occur when the EMT has the correct intent but does not carry out an action as intended, such as mistakenly using the wrong piece of equipment. Mistakes occur when the EMT has an incorrect intention that leads to incorrect action.
- Rules-based: The EMT incorrectly applies a rule, applies a bad or wrong rule, or fails to apply the correct rules. For example, an EMT is injured because of failing to assess safety before approaching a patient.
- Knowledge-based: The EMT's knowledge is not adequate for the situation.

EMS personnel can help reduce errors by debriefing, constantly reevaluating and questioning assumptions, using established protocols and decision aids, and asking for assistance when needed.

Continuous Quality Improvement (CQI)

Continuous quality improvement (CQI) emphasizes the organization and systems and processes within that organization rather than emphasizing individuals. It recognizes internal customers (staff) and external customers (patients) and uses data to improve processes. CQI represents the concept that most processes can be improved. CQI uses the scientific method of experimentation to meet needs and improve services and uses various tools, such as brainstorming, multivoting, various charts and diagrams, storyboarding, and meetings. Core concepts include the following:

- Quality and success are meeting or exceeding internal and external customers' needs and expectations.
- Problems relate to processes, and variations in processes lead to variations in results.
- Change can be made in small steps.

Steps to CQI include the following:

- Forming a knowledgeable team.
- Identifying and defining measures used to determine success.
- Brainstorming strategies for change.
- Plan, collect, and use data as part of making decisions.
- Test changes and revise or refine as needed.

Research

Research is especially important in identifying the need for changes in procedures and protocols in order to improve patient outcomes. Research depends on the gathering of data. Data collection may include direct observations, surveys, interviews, and various other sources of information, such as documents and audiovisual materials. Literature research requires a comprehensive evaluation of current (≤5 years) and/or historical information. Most literature research begins with an Internet search of databases, which provides listings of books, journals, and other materials on specific topics. Databases vary in content, and many contain only a reference listing with or without an abstract, so once the listing is obtained, the researcher must do a further search (publisher, library, etc.) to locate the material. Some databases require a subscription, but access is often available through educational or healthcare institutions. In order to search effectively, the researcher should begin by writing a brief explanation of the research to help identify possible keywords and synonyms to use as search words.

Evidence-Based Decision Making

Although traditional medical practice has been based on knowledge, intuition, and judgment, these practices have not always been supported by evidence. **Evidence-based decision making** results in best practices based on best evidence. Steps include the following:

- Formulating a question regarding treatment and/or procedures.
- Conducting a search of the appropriate medical literature, often beginning with the search of an online database to find research that is related to the question.
- Determining the validity (measure of accuracy) and reliability (consistency) of the evidence. Evaluating the level of evidence (1a and 1b are the most valid, and 1c is required by state or federal regulations or is an industry standard).
- Assessing data (information) to determine if they apply to current needs.
- Drawing up a plan for change with input from all staff members.

- Implementing changes.
- Monitoring changes and outcomes.

Methods of Data Collection

When developing **data collection procedures** to determine needs, the following must be considered: the purpose of the data collection, the audience for which the data are intended, the types of questions to be answered, the scope of the research, and the resources available to carry out data collection.

Method	Issues regarding procedures
Direct observation	Observers must be selected and trained on how to observe and when and how to record observations.
Interviews	Interview questions must be developed and validated, and the interviewers must be given practice time.
Questionnaires	The type of questionnaire, the questions, and the Likert scale must be determined as well as the method of distribution (one-on-one, group, email, Internet).
Record review	A form or checklist should be developed to guide record review, and the records should be selected based on criteria established for the research.
Secondary analysis	The databases to be mined should be selected, and the criteria for the research should be established, including keywords, time frames, and populations.

Personal Protective Equipment (PPE)

Personal protective equipment (PPE) should be readily available in the appropriate sizes for each EMS individual.

- Gowns: Should be worn for risk of splash or spray with body fluids (severe bleeding, childbirth) and should be fluid resistant.
- Eye protectors: Should be worn for risk of splash or spray with body fluids or contact with debris, such as at a worksite or in a collapsing building. Goggles should fit snugly and have antifog features. (Prescription eyeglasses do not take the place of goggles.)
- Face shields: Provide protection for face, eyes, nose, and mouth. These are preferred to goggles when there is risk of spray or splash of body fluids. They should wrap around and cover the forehead and extend to below the chin.
- Masks: Protect the nose and mouth from fluids and particles and should be fluid resistant, fit snugly, and have a flexible nosepiece.
- Respirators (such as N95, N99, and N100): Protect the nose, mouth, and airway passages exposed to hazardous or infectious aerosols, including bacteria (tuberculosis [TB], measles patients).

Hand Hygiene and Gloves

Hand hygiene should be done before eating, before and after direct contact with a patient's skin, after contact with any body fluids, after contact with inanimate objects in the patient's immediate vicinity, when moving hands from a dirty to a clean area, after removing gloves, and after using the restroom.

Hand hygiene is carried out in the following two manners:

- Antiseptic soaps/detergents: For visible soiling, after exposure to diarrhea stool or a patient with diarrhea, before eating, and after using the restroom. Wet hands, apply product, rub hands together vigorously for 15 seconds, covering all surfaces, rinse hands with water, and use a disposable towel to dry them.
- Alcohol-based hand sanitizers (the most effective way to kill bacteria): For all other situations. Apply product and rub hands together, including between the fingers, for about 20 seconds until the skin surfaces are dry.

Gloves must be worn when touching any body fluids, nonintact skin, open wounds, or mucous membranes (eyes, mouth, nose); gloves should be changed when moving from a dirty area to a clean one or from one patient to another.

Procedures for Exposure/Contamination

Any **exposure/contamination** should be reported at hand-off and to the appropriate infection control person following protocols, and follow-up care should be sought if necessary. Decontamination procedures are as follows:

- <u>Skin:</u> Cleanse the area thoroughly with soap and water.
- <u>Eyes:</u> Flush with water for 20 minutes.
- <u>Needlestick:</u> Wash the area with soap and water and report immediately.
- <u>Clothing:</u> Remove the clothing as soon as possible, and wash visible soiling of skin with soap and water if a shower is not immediately available, but shower as soon as possible. Clothes should be washed separately in a washing machine at the workplace.
- <u>Equipment/Vehicle:</u> Clean thoroughly with disinfectant. Dispose of equipment if unable to adequately decontaminate it.

When reporting exposures/contamination, note the type of exposure, the date and time of exposure, circumstances, actions taken to decontaminate, and any other required information.

Isolation Guidelines

The **2007 CDC Guideline for Isolation Precautions** includes the standard precautions that apply to all patients and transmission-based precautions for those with known or suspected infections. **Standard precautions** should be used for all patients because all body fluids (sweat, urine, feces, blood, and sputum) and nonintact skin and mucous membranes may be infected.

Hand hygiene	Wash hands before and after each patient contact and after any contact with body fluids and contaminated items. Use soap and water for visible soiling.
Protective equipment	Use personal protective equipment (PPE), such as gloves, gowns, and masks, eye protection, and/or face shields, when anticipating contact with body fluids or contaminated skin.
Respiratory hygiene/ Cough etiquette	Use source-control measures, such as covering cough, disposing of tissues, using a surgical mask on the person coughing or on staff to prevent inhalation of droplets, and properly disposing of dressings and used equipment. Wash hands after contacting respiratory secretions. Maintain a distance of >3 feet from a coughing person when possible.
Sharps	Dispose of sharps, such as needles, carefully in sharps containers. Do not recap needles.

Transmission-Based Precautions

The **2007 CDC Guideline for Isolation Precautions** includes the standard precautions that apply to all patients and **transmission-based precautions** for those with known or suspected infections as well as those with excessive wound drainage, other discharge, or fecal incontinence. Transmission-based precautions include the following:

Contact	Use PPE, including gown and gloves, for all contacts with the patient or the patient's immediate environment.
Droplet	(Appropriate for influenza, streptococcus infection, pertussis, rhinovirus, and adenovirus and pathogens that remain viable and infectious for only short distances.) Use a mask while caring for the patient. Maintain the patient at a distance of >3 feet away from other patients (with a curtain separating them in an emergency department). Use a patient mask if transporting a patient.
Airborne	(Appropriate for measles, chickenpox, tuberculosis, and severe acute respiratory syndrome [SARS] because pathogens remain viable and infectious for long distances.) Use ≥N95 respirators (or masks) while caring for the patient. The patient should be placed in an airborne infection isolation room in an emergency department.

Immunizations for EMS Personnel

The Centers for Disease Control and Prevention (CDC) recommends the following **immunizations** for all healthcare workers, including EMS personnel:

- Hepatitis B: Three-dose series (now, in one month, and five months later) followed by an anti-HBs serologic test 30 to 60 days after the third immunization.
- Measles, mumps, rubella (MMR): Two-dose series with the second immunization at least 28 days after the first for those born during or after 1957 and those born before 1957 without proof of immunity.
- Varicella (chickenpox): Two doses, four weeks apart. (A combined MMRV immunization is available.)
- Influenza: Annually.
- Tetanus, diphtheria, and pertussis (Tdap): One time with a tetanus (TD) booster every 10 years. The TD injection does not protect against pertussis (whooping cough).
- Meningococcal: One dose.

Screening for tuberculosis with a chest x-ray or skin test is also recommended.

Stress

The EMT must often deal with **stressful incidents**, such as dangerous situations (storm conditions, gunshots, falling debris); critically ill patients; unpleasant sights, sounds, and odors; multipatient incidents; and angry/upset patients, family members, and bystanders. The EMT should not argue or become defensive but should remain calm and supportive, allowing the patient to express his or her feelings and trying to defuse the situation while administering medical care and cooperating with other first responders. If a patient has no pulse or respirations and does not have a valid do-not-resuscitate (DNR) order, the EMT should attempt resuscitation unless doing so puts the EMT at risk; the injuries are not compatible with life; or obvious signs of death are present, such as tissue decay, livor mortis, which is discoloration in the lowermost blood vessels from pooled blood shortly after death, or rigor mortis, which is stiffening of the joints that occurs within 2 to 6 hours of death (verified by checking two or more joints). After 24 to 48 hours of rigor mortis, the muscles become flaccid.

Warning signs of stress often begin with difficulty sleeping and nightmares about work, loss of appetite, and lack of interest in usual activities, including work and intimacy. The individual may feel increasingly sad and depressed and may have difficulty concentrating, making decisions, and carrying out tasks. The individual may also begin to isolate from others and exhibit irritability with coworkers, family, and friends. Some individuals develop physical symptoms related to stress, such as stomach upset, headaches, nausea, and high blood pressure (BP), whereas others may experience panic attacks. Some individuals may try to self-medicate with alcohol or drugs. When experiencing the warning signs of stress, the individual should talk about the problems with someone trusted, such as a physician, coworker, supervisor, or family member, and he or she may need to seek assistance from a professional counselor. Lifestyle changes, such as decreasing the use of alcohol or drugs, exercising regularly, and practicing relaxation exercises, may help to relieve stress.

Stress reactions include the following:

- Acute stress reaction: This reaction usually occurs quickly (minutes to hours) in response to an event that is stressful (such as the death of a child or a multiple-casualty incident). The individual may experience physical symptoms (with the release of adrenaline) such as rapid pulse, nausea, chest tightness, headache, fast respirations, and increased perspiration. An acute stress reaction usually recedes quickly, but it may persist for weeks in some individuals.
- Delayed stress reaction: Although the individual may cope well with a stressful event initially, months later, the person may begin to have nightmares, anxiety, and other indications of post-traumatic stress.
- Cumulative stress reaction: This type of stress reaction occurs when the individual has repeated stressors (either in the workplace or in his or her personal life) that cause repeated acute stress reactions, resulting in various physical and psychological problems. This is especially common in EMS personnel.

Prevention of Response-Related Injuries

Prevention of response-related injuries includes the following:

- Infectious diseases: Use PPE and understand the spread of infectious diseases—air (coughing), direct contact (blood, vomitus, other body fluids), needlestick, contaminated food/equipment, and sexual transmission. Maintain current immunizations.
- Personal habits: Obtain adequate sleep, nutrition, and exercise. Avoid excessive alcohol and tobacco.
- Environmental hazards: Conduct a 360° assessment. Note traffic hazards, the vehicle's condition, fire, leaking fluids, downed power lines, hazardous materials (look for placards and warning symbols; avoid the area until it is cleared). Use PPE and respirators as indicated.
- Violence: Defuse situations, make a safe response (assistance of law enforcement), and use restraints if necessary for dangerous or violent individuals.
- Collisions: Drive safely; avoid speeding and driving through stop signs and red lights when possible. Wear seat belts and/or safety harnesses.

End of Life/Death and Dying

Grief is a normal response to the death or severe illness/abnormality of a patient. How a person deals with grief is very personal, and each will grieve differently. Elisabeth Kübler-Ross identified **five stages of grief**, which can apply to patients and family members. A person may not go through each stage, but he or she usually goes through two of the five stages.

Stage	Patient/Family	Appropriate EMT response
1. Denial	Resistive to information, stunned, immobile, detached, unable to respond appropriately	Be patient and supportive and repeat information as needed.
2. Anger	Lashing out, overt hostility, self-blame, blaming others	Do not respond in anger or take statements personally; remain calm and supportive, but be alert to the risk of physical attack.
3. Bargaining	If–then thinking, demanding another opinion or expert, praying	Avoid making any judgmental statements.
4. Depression	Tearful, crying, withdrawn, sad, isolated	Encourage expression of feelings, remain supportive, and assure the individual that these feelings are normal.
5. Acceptance	Resolution	Listen patiently and remain supportive.

Signs and Symbols

Sign/Symbol	Interpretation
	Flame: Includes flammable materials and gases and those that are self-heating or self-reactive.
	Corrosion: Includes substances that can cause skin burns, metal corrosion, and eye damage.
	Health hazard: Includes carcinogens, toxic substances, and respiratory irritants.
	Poison: Includes materials, gases, or substances that are extremely toxic and may result in death or severe illness.

	Irritant: Includes material, gases, or substances that are irritants to skin, eyes, and/or respiratory tract, are acutely toxic, or have a narcotic effect.
	Biohazard: Includes biological substances, such as body fluids, that pose a threat to humans. Appears on sharps containers that hold contaminated needles.

Principles of Body Mechanics

Basic principles of body mechanics include the following:

- Avoid reaching for prolonged periods of time, overhead, or more than 20 inches away.
- Avoid pulling—push, roll, or slide instead.
- Avoid lifting—push, roll, or slide instead.
- Lift with leg muscles, not with the back.
- Hold weight close to the body rather than at arm's length.
- Flex at the hips and knees, not the waist.
- Carry patients head first upstairs and feet first downstairs.
- Maintain a straight back and avoid twisting.
- Assess weight and recognize limitations in lifting/carrying.
- Get help when necessary, and communicate every step with your partner ("Lift on the count of three").
- Maintain a firm base of support with feet apart (shoulder width) to stabilize your stance.
- Maintain the line of gravity (the imaginary line between your center of gravity and the ground) within the base of support.
- Position yourself close to an object that is to be lifted or carried.
- Lift patients from stable ground.

Moving and Lifting Patients

Techniques for moving patients include the following:

- <u>Direct ground lift:</u> Use only for lightweight individuals with no suspected spinal injuries. Three rescuers line up on one side of the patient, and each kneels on the same knee. The EMT at the head places one arm under the patient's neck and shoulder and the other arm under the patient's lower back. The middle EMT places his or her arms above and below the patient's waist, and the EMT at the patient's feet places his or her arms under the knees and lower legs. On the count of three, they roll the patient onto their knees and toward their chests. On the count of three, they stand and move the patient.
- <u>Power lift:</u> Place feet (shoulder width) apart and pointing slightly outward; tighten the back and abdominal muscles. Squat down as though sitting. Place hands 10 inches apart with the palms upward (power grip) while grasping the stretcher and lift with the upper body becoming vertical before the hips rise.

- Extremity lift: Requires two EMTs. One EMT squats at the patient's head and another is at one side by the patient's knees. The EMT at the head folds the patient's arms across the chest and grasps the patient by wrapping both arms around the torso under the patient's arms and grasping the patient's wrists. The second EMT slides his or her hands beneath the patient's knees and lower legs, and together they stand and lift the patient.
- Squat lift: Requires two EMTs. One EMT squats with the back straight and the weak foot slightly forward at the head of patient, and the other EMT is in the same position at the patient's feet. Grasp the patient's upper body as for the extremity lift and grasp the patient's feet. Both EMTs push up with the stronger foot and lift with the upper body becoming vertical before the hips rise.
- Logroll: Used to position carrying devices under the patient and for some transfers; it requires two EMTs positioned on the same side of the patient. Place the patient's arm on the side that he or she is being turned to above his or her head or over the chest. Place the patient's other arm across his or her chest. If on the ground, squat close to the patient. The EMT at the patient's head reaches across the patient and grasps his or her shoulders and trunk while the second EMT grasps his or her trunk and legs. On the count of three, they turn the patient in one smooth move.
- Draw-sheet transfer: Requires four EMTs with two positioned on one side of the patient and two positioned on the other side but on the opposite side of the bed or stretcher to which the patient will be transferred. The logroll technique is used to place a draw sheet under the patient. EMTs on both sides roll the edges of the draw sheet until the edges are close to the patient. On the count of three, they lift the patient slightly and move the patient across to the bed.

Backboards and Cervical Collars

Backboards were originally designed to transfer patients. However, **backboards and cervical collars** have been routinely used for EMS rescues for many years without evidence-based studies supporting their use. The premise was that stabilizing the spine and neck would prevent further injury in case a spinal injury had occurred, but spinal injuries are relatively rare, and some studies indicate that these devices do not provide any protection and, in fact, may cause damage. Additionally, cervical collars restrict the airway by 20% or more and may worsen injuries if not properly sized for the patient. Because of these findings, some EMS no longer routinely use backboards but use a vacuum mattress in a scoop basket instead. The American Association of Neurological Surgeons/Congress of Neurological Surgeons (AANS/CNS) guidelines advise that spinal immobilization using a backboard be reserved for known or suspected spinal cord injury without penetrating injury, although the use of the cervical collar is still recommended until the cervical spine is assessed for injury. Short backboards may be used to support a patient's back in a sitting position.

Restraints

Restraints should be avoided if possible, although if a combative patient poses a risk to him- or herself or EMS personnel, restraints may be necessary to safely assess, treat, and transport the patient, keeping in mind that the altered state of consciousness may result from drug or alcohol use; traumatic injury; or from a mental or physical disorder, such as schizophrenia, dementia, or hypoglycemia (insulin reaction). Protocols for use of restraints must be followed, and restraints should be applied under medical direction. If possible, the police should be present and there should be one EMS personnel for each limb, staying beyond the limb's range of motion until ready to secure the limb, with one EMT talking to the patient and explaining the procedure. The EMT should avoid unnecessary force, which may result in increased combativeness and injury to the patient or others. Patients should not be restrained in the prone (face-down) position. Documentation must include the reason for restraining the patient, the time, and the method of restraint.

Common **types of physical restraints** include the following:

- Soft: Padded cuffs (often leather) that fasten about the wrists and ankles and are attached to a long board. These are the most commonly used restraints.
- Stretcher/Spinal board straps: These may be strapped across the chest (not too tight), abdomen, or legs to help restrict movement.
- Long board/Spinal board: Patient should be restrained to the long board and then placed on a wheeled stretcher and never tied to or fastened to the stretcher.
- Spit sock: A hood that fits over the patient's head to prevent him or her from biting or spitting.
- Cervical collar: This is used to protect the patient's cervical spine and to prevent him or her from biting.

The EMT should not place the patient in handcuffs or hard plastic ties. If these were placed on a patient by a law enforcement officer and must stay in place, such as with a criminal or an extremely violent patient, then a law enforcement officer must stay with the patient at all times.

Emergency Moves

Emergency moves may be needed if the patient and/or EMT is in immediate danger from fire, explosives, or other hazards; if the patient requires life-saving treatment, such as cardiopulmonary resuscitation (CPR); or if the patient is in water, such as a pond or lake. Emergency moves include the following:

- Blanket drag: Logroll the patient onto a blanket, wrap the patient in the blanket, grasp the blanket near the patient's head while in a squatting position with your back straight, and drag. If there are two rescuers, the other should be positioned at the patient's feet and should be pushing.
- Clothing drag: Squat down by the patient's head, securely grasp the clothing near the patient's neck or shoulders (avoid grasping by a T-shirt), and drag the patient.
- Arm drag: Squat down by the patient's head. Fold the patient's arms across his or her chest. Grasp the patient under the arms, wrapping your arms about the torso and grasping the patient's wrists to stabilize his or her arms. Drag the patient.

Urgent moves, such as with altered mental status, shock, or breathing difficulties, should also be done as quickly as possible.

Emergency moves can be carried out by one rescuer if no other assistance is available, as follows:

- Firefighter's drag: Tie the patient's wrists together with any available material. Straddle the patient and pull the patient's arms over your neck and then crawl forward, dragging him or her beneath you.

- Firefighter's carry: Grasp the patient's knees and pull them together and up. Stand on the patient's feet and reach out and grab one of the patient's arms with one hand. Pull the patient upright, and, as the patient elevates, place your other hand between the patient's legs. Place the patient's arm behind your neck and continue to pull the patient and lift until he or she is draped across your upper back with the arm hanging free. Then grasp the patient's arm that is hanging with the hand that is between the legs to secure the patient.

Minimum Data Sets

Minimum data sets are the minimum data specifically required for EMS services. These consist of the following:

- Patient information: This derives from the assessment including the patient's primary complaint and the findings during the initial assessment—the patient's name and address; vital signs (blood pressure [BP], pulse [P], and respiration rate [R]); and descriptions of any wounds, injuries, pain, or other symptoms. The patient's demographics (age, gender, ethnic background) should be noted as well as any other identifying or essential information.
- Administrative information: This includes the time of the initial report, time the EMS unit was notified, time of arrival at the incident, time of leaving the scene, time of arrival at the destination (hospital, trauma center), and time of hand-off.
- Accurate/Synchronous clocks: All members of the EMS system should use accurate and synchronous clocks so that they all are set to the same time to ensure there is no disparity in time reporting.

Prehospital Care Report

The **prehospital care report** serves as a legal document to show that emergent care was provided. It describes the condition of the patient upon the EMT's arrival at the scene, interventions provided, and changes in the patient's condition; it is essential to ensure continuity of care. The documenting EMT may be called in to legal proceedings. The prehospital care report may also be used for educational purposes, such as through debriefing and case review. Additionally, the report is used administratively as the basis for billing as well as for the collection of data for research and evaluation of continuous quality improvement. Required elements of documentation include the time of events (receipt of call, arrival at incident, time of transport, arrival at destination), assessment findings (vital signs, injuries, bleeding, mental status), emergent care, changes in the patient's condition, response to the treatment provided, scene observations (specific place/area), hazards, and disposition of patient (care refusal, transportation, hand-off). Documentation may be on paper or may be done electronically and may combine checkboxes and narrative reports. Run data are those data elements that are required for reporting of each run.

Narrative Documentation

With **narrative documentation,** the EMT should take care not to repeat the same information already provided in checkboxes. The EMT should describe what was observed directly rather than the conclusions based on those observations and should record all pertinent information and observations, avoiding nonstandardized abbreviations and radio codes, which may be misunderstood or misinterpreted. Any pertinent negatives, such as patient or family complaints, must be documented. If the incident has legal implications, such as in the case of assault, any pertinent comments or sensitive information ("I was raped") should be quoted directly and the source should be noted. Care should be taken to write clearly and spell correctly. Time should be documented for every intervention and reassessment. Any state or local reporting requirements must be met in documentation, and the contents of the prehospital report should remain confidential and be distributed only to appropriate healthcare providers. No data may be falsified, and any errors and steps taken to correct those errors must be documented.

Patient Refusal of Medical Care

According to the **Patient Self-Determination Act** (1990), competent patients have the right to refuse any medical treatment, and parents have the right to make this decision for minor children. If a patient refuses care, then the EMT should try to persuade the patient to go to the hospital by giving the reasons and possible consequences of refusal. The patient should be asked to sign the refusal form, and a family member, police officer, or bystander should sign as a witness to the patient's signing or witness the patient's refusal to sign. The EMT should complete documentation of any assessment carried out and any refusal of the patient to assessment. The EMT should carefully document the conversation between the EMT and patient regarding refusal of care and consequences and should document the proposed care as well as the information the EMT gave the patient about alternate care (such as a visit to the personal physician) and the willingness to return if the patient has a change of mind.

Special Situations

Documentation errors: In handwritten documents, draw one line through the error, initial, and write the correct information beside the error. If information was omitted, add a note with the date and your initials. If documentation was electronic, follow the method prescribed for corrections.

Multiple-casualty incidents: Record information temporarily for later complete documentation, if necessary, following the procedures in place for such an incident.

Incident reports: Fill out forms as soon as possible, document any witnesses to the incident, and file forms according to protocol. Incident reports are often maintained separately from prehospital reports.

Special-situation reports: Used for events/incidents that must be reported to an outside authority or as a supplement to the prehospital report. Fill out the report as soon as possible, and include the names of all parties involved; use objective descriptions, and avoid stating conclusions. Maintain a personal copy.

Transfer reports: Ensure that they contain minimum data sets and provide a transfer signature. These are used during hand-off.

EMS System Communication

With the **EMT's arrival** at the scene of an incident, he or she should assess the situation and the need for added resources, such as additional EMS personnel or police, and contact the appropriate authorities to request assistance. When additional EMS personnel arrive or contact is made with medical control or the receiving facility, the EMT should self-identify and provide a verbal report of the patient's current condition, including demographic information such as age and gender. The EMT should report the patient's chief complaint and provide any history that is pertinent as well as the condition of the patient on arrival and any history of major illnesses. The EMT should also report the results of the patient assessment, including the vital signs and any physical/psychological findings, as well as any treatment provided and the patient's response to the treatment. The EMT should communicate with law enforcement officers and other responders, such as firefighters, especially regarding safety concerns.

Components of an EMS communication system include the base station of a two-way radio system, which is in a fixed location, such as a dispatch center. The base station facilitates communication among a number of hand-held/mobile radios. There is often only one channel per base station, so additional base stations may be installed to add more channels. Radio transmitters/receivers may be vehicular mounted or mobile, although mobile transmitters/receivers may have limited range because they tend to have lower power (1–5 watts) than do base stations (20–50 watts). Typically, the mobile device has a range of 10– preserve evidence15 miles over average terrain, but it is shorter in rugged terrain. The Federal Communications Commission (FCC) controls radio frequencies, and those used for EMS are in the public safety pool.

Communication with Medical Control

The EMT may be in **communication with medical control** regarding a patient's condition and need for medication. Medical control may be at the receiving facility or at a separate site. Upon receiving an order by phone or radio, the EMT should repeat back the order and dosage to ensure that the message was received correctly. When using the radio, the radio must be turned on and the press-to-talk (PTT) button must be pressed before beginning transmission. The EMT should address the medical control person by name and give the name of the EMT's unit. Transmissions should be brief and to the point, avoiding unnecessary pleasantries, codes, agency-specific terms, profanity, and meaningless phrases, keeping in mind that the airways are public. The EMT should give individual digits for long numbers, use "affirmative" and "negative" in place of "yes" and "no," and say "over" when the transmission is finished. Reports should be objective rather than opinion based and should avoid offering a diagnosis. The dispatcher must be notified when the unit leaves the scene.

Phone/Cellular Communication and Interpersonal Communication with Patients

Phone/Cellular communication: This is similar to radio communication, but the EMT should be familiar with important phone numbers (such as medical control, hospitals, trauma centers) or have the numbers prominently posted for access. The EMT should also be aware of dead spots that may prevent communication and should have a backup plan (radio) for when cellular transmission fails.

Interpersonal communication: Upon arrival at the scene of an incident, the EMT should self-introduce, making eye contact, and he or she should communicate using language that the patient can understand, that is age-appropriate, and that avoids any medical jargon. The EMT should be positioned at or below the level of the patient if possible to avoid intimidating the patient and should remain aware of body language. The EMT should be honest and speak slowly and calmly, using the patient's first or last name, depending on the age of the patient and the circumstances. The EMT may request interpreters if necessary.

Effective Communication and Interviewing Techniques

Effective communication begins with a self-introduction and an introduction of other team members to the patient and family and includes respecting the patient's privacy by shielding the patient from passersby if possible and avoiding loudly repeating any patient information. If possible, the EMT should adjust lighting and limit outside distractions such as noise. When interviewing the patient, the EMT should ask open-ended questions (such as "Can you describe your pain?") and avoid questions that can be answered with "yes" or "no." The EMT should ask direct questions, such as "When did the pain start?" Questions should be asked one at a time while allowing the patient/family time to respond. It's especially important to observe the patient's body language (posture, eye contact, gestures, and tone of voice) to determine if it matches his or her words and to avoid medical/professional jargon. The EMT should avoid giving false reassurances or advice and should avoid leading/biased questions, being too talkative, interrupting the patient, and asking "why" questions, such as "Why did you take an overdose of medication?"

Special Interview Situations

Interviewing **hostile patients** requires a calm response, avoiding negative responses and using reflective statements, such as "I can understand your feelings." The EMT should maintain eye contact (50% to 60% of the time) and try to defuse the situation, but he or she should avoid staring or standing too close and having crossed arms because this may be misinterpreted as threatening behavior. If patients are **sexually aggressive**, it's important to tell them that the behavior is inappropriate and to ask them to stop. When interviewing patients under the **influence of drugs or alcohol,** try to ask essential questions such as the type and amount of drug/alcohol ingested. Obtain information from family or friends if necessary. When patients are **hearing impaired**, the EMT should face the person directly, speak slowly and distinctly (but avoid shouting), provide information in writing if possible, use pantomime, and try to reduce environmental noise. Knowledge of the alphabet in sign language can be very useful to communicate with the deaf, especially if a sign-language translator is unavailable.

When **interviewing elderly patients**, the EMT should be alert to possible cognitive, hearing, or vision impairments, especially if the patient appears confused upon questioning or his or her answers are inappropriate. The EMT should ask if the patient has eyeglasses or a hearing aid and should obtain them if possible. The patient's family may be able to assist with the interview. If the patient's speech is unclear, he or she may need to put in dentures. When communicating with a **pediatric patient**, the EMT should have the parent or caregiver comfort the child and answer questions, especially if the child is an infant or is very young. The EMT should use simple sentences and age-appropriate language and explain to the child what he or she is doing to help alleviate the child's fear. Adolescents should be addressed directly even if a parent or caregiver is providing some information, and, in some cases, the adolescent will provide more information if the parent/caregiver is not present.

Dynamics of the Communication Process

The **communication process**, which includes the sender-receiver feedback loop, is based on Claude Shannon's article, "A Mathematical Theory of Communication" (1948), in which he provided the basis for information theory and described three necessary steps of successful communication: encoding a message, transmitting it through a channel, and decoding it. The resultant communication process begins with the sender, who serves as the encoder and determines the content of the message. The medium is the form the message takes (digital, written, audiovisual), and the channel is the method of delivery (mail, radio, TV, phone, email, text message). The recipient (receiver), who acts as the decoder, determines the meaning from the message. Feedback helps to determine whether or not the communication is successful and whether the message is understood as intended. This process is referred to as the sender-receiver feedback loop. Context is the environment (physical and psychological) in which the communication occurs, and interference is any factor that impacts the communication process. Interference may be external (such as environmental noise) or internal (such as emotional distress or anxiety).

Therapeutic Communication

Therapeutic communication begins with respect for the individual/family and the assumption that all communication, verbal and nonverbal, has meaning. Listening must be done empathetically. Techniques that facilitate communication include the following:

Introduction	Make a personal introduction and use the individual's name: "Mrs. Brown, I am Toby Williams, your EMT."
Encouragement	Use an open-ended opening question: "Is there anything you'd like to discuss?" Acknowledge comments: Say "yes" and "I understand." Allow silence and observe nonverbal behavior rather than trying to force a conversation. Ask for clarification if the patient's statements are unclear. Reflect the patient's statements back (use sparingly): Individual: "I hate this hospital." EMT: "You hate this hospital?"
Empathy	Make observations: "You are shaking," and "You seem worried." Recognize feelings: Individual: "I want to get well." EMT: "It must be hard for you to deal with this illness." Provide information as honestly and completely as possible about the patient's condition, treatment, and procedures and respond to the individual's questions and concerns.
Exploration	Verbally express implied messages: Individual: "This treatment is too much trouble." EMT: "Do you think the treatment isn't helping you?" Explore a topic, but allow the individual to terminate the discussion without further probing: "I'd like to hear how you feel about that."
Orientation	Indicate reality: Individual: "Someone is screaming." EMT: "That sound was a police siren." Comment on distortions without directly agreeing or disagreeing: Individual: "That policeman promised I could go to St. John's Hospital." EMT: "Really? That's surprising because this ambulance is based at County Hospital."

Collaboration	Work together to achieve better results: "Maybe if we talk about this, we can figure out a way to make the treatment easier for you."
Validation	Seek validation: "Do you feel better now?" or "Did the medication help you breathe better?"

Cultural Considerations

Hmong	The eldest male in the family makes the decisions for the family and is deferred to by other family members, so the EMT should ask who should receive information about the patient. Communication should be polite and respectful, avoiding direct eye contact, which is considered rude. Disagreeing is considered rude, so "yes" may mean "I hear you" and NOT "I agree with you."
Mexican	Mexican culture perceives time with more flexibility than does American culture, so if patients/family need to be present at a particular time, the EMT should specify the exact time ("be here at 1:30 PM") and explain the reason rather than saying something that is more vague, such as "be here after lunch." People may appear to be unassertive or unable to make decisions when they are simply showing respect to the EMT by being deferent. In traditional families, the males make decisions, so a woman may wait for the husband or other males in the family to make decisions about her treatment or care.
Middle Eastern	In Middle Eastern countries, males make the decisions, so issues for discussion or decision should be directed to males, such as the patient's spouse or son, and males may be direct in stating what they want, sometimes appearing demanding. Middle Easterners often require less personal space and may stand very close. If a male EMT must care for a female patient, then the family should be advised that only medical treatments, not personal care, will be done by the male EMT.
Asian	Asian families may expect the EMT to remain authoritative and to give directions and may not question the EMT's authority. Disagreeing is considered impolite. "Yes" may only mean that the person is heard, not that they agree with the person. When asked if they understand, they may indicate that they do even when they clearly do not so as not to offend the EMT. Asians may avoid eye contact as an indication of respect.

Cultural Competence

There are a number of issues related to cultural competence in communicating with others.

- **Eye contact:** Many cultures use eye contact differently than what is common in the United States. Some patients and families, such as Asians, Native Americans, and Arabs, may avoid direct eye contact, considering it rude, or they may look away to signal disapproval or may look down to signal respect. Careful observation of the way family members use eye contact can help to determine what will be most comfortable for the patient/family.

- **Distance**: Some cultures stand close to others (<4 feet) when speaking (Middle Easterners, Hispanics), and others stand at a greater distance (>4 feet) (Northern Europeans, many Americans). There is a considerable difference relating to concepts of personal space among cultures. Allowing the family to approach or observing whether they tend to move closer, lean forward, or move back can help to determine a comfortable distance for communication.
- **Time**: Americans tend to be time oriented, and they expect people to be on time, but time is viewed more flexibly in many other cultures.

Interviewing Techniques

If possible, the patient should be interviewed alone or should be asked if he or she wants family members present. Verbal and nonverbal responses should be observed during **an interview.** Information should include not only the patient's facts but also the patient's attitude and concerns. The EMT should ask one question at a time in language that the patient understands and avoid providing false reassurances and advice or interrupting. Strategies include the following:

- Ask open-ended informational questions (as opposed to yes/no) with "who," "what," "where," "when," and "how," but avoid questions with "why" if possible.
  - Instead of "Why do you continue to use heroin?" ask "Have you tried to quit drug use?"
- Ask brief clarifying questions: "How long have you had weakness in your left side?"
- Provide a list of options: "Is your headache throbbing, stabbing, or dull?"
- Rephrase/reflect to encourage clarification.
  - Patient: "My husband had the same type of fall and died a month later."
  - EMT: "You're afraid you might die from this fall."

Conditions for Consent

The **conditions for consent** for care and decision-making capacity include the following:

- 18 years or older: Patients who are younger may have the right to give consent for all or some medical treatment in some states. State laws vary; for example, the age of consent for medical treatment in Alabama is 14.
- Mentally competent to make decisions: May be impaired by mental disability, injury, illness, or substance abuse (intoxication).
- Court-emancipated minor.
- Military service.
- Marriage.

Consent may be expressed if the patient is able to give informed consent, or it may be implied, such as when care is provided in an emergent situation in which the patient is unable to give consent. Parents or caregivers give consent for minors younger than the age of 18 unless they have been emancipated. If parents or caregivers are unavailable to give consent, life-saving emergent care, general medical assessment, and medical care to prevent further injury or harm can be provided without consent.

Informed Consent

Patients or their families must provide **informed consent** for all treatments that they receive. This includes a thorough explanation of all procedures and treatment and the associated risks. Patients/families should be apprised of all options and allowed input on the type of treatments.

Patients/families should be apprised of all reasonable risks and any complications that might be life threatening or increase morbidity. The American Medical Association has established guidelines for informed consent as follows:

- Explanation of the diagnosis.
- Nature of and reason for the treatment or procedure.
- Risks and benefits.
- Alternative options (regardless of cost or insurance coverage).
- Risks and benefits of alternative options.
- Risks and benefits of not having a treatment or procedure.
- Providing informed consent is a requirement of all states.

The requirement for informed consent may be waived in life-threatening situations and if the EMT cannot obtain informed consent because the patient cannot communicate and legal consent cannot be obtained.

Health Insurance Portability and Accountability Act of 1996 (HIPAA)

Sensitive information is classified under the **Health Insurance Portability and Accountability Act of 1996** (HIPAA) as protected health information (PHI), and it includes the following:

- Any information about an individual's past, present, or future health or condition (mental or physical).
- Provision of health care.
- Any identifying information related to payment for healthcare services.
- Identifying information: Name, address, Social Security number, birth date, and any document or material that contains the identifying information.

Personal information can be shared with a spouse, legal guardians, those with durable power of attorney for the patient, and those involved in the care of the patient, such as physicians, without a specific release. HIPAA mandates the following privacy and security rules to ensure that health information and individual privacy are protected:

- Privacy rule: Protected information includes any information included in the medical record (electronic or paper), conversations between the doctor and other healthcare providers, billing information, and any other form of health information.
- Security rule: Any electronic health information must be secure and protected against threats, hazards, or nonpermitted disclosure.

Advance Directives, Durable Power of Attorney, and Do-Not-Resuscitate (DNR) Order

In accordance with federal and state laws, individuals have the right to self-determination in health care, including decisions about end-of-life care through **advance directives** such as living wills and the right to assign a surrogate person to make decisions through a **durable power of attorney**. Patients should routinely be questioned about an advanced directive because they may present at a healthcare organization without the document. Patients who have indicated that they desire a **do-not-resuscitate (DNR) order** should not receive resuscitative treatments for terminal illness or conditions in which meaningful recovery cannot occur. Patients and families of those with terminal illnesses should be questioned as to whether the patients are hospice patients. For those with DNR requests or those withdrawing life support, staff should provide the patient palliative rather than curative measures, such as pain control and/or oxygen, and emotional support to the patient and family. Religious traditions and beliefs about death should be treated with respect.

Patient Refusal of Medical Care

According to the **Patient Self-Determination Act** (1990), competent patients have the right to **refusal of care,** and parents have the right to make this decision for minor children. If a patient refuses care, then the EMT should try to persuade the patient to go to the hospital by giving the reasons and possible consequences of refusal. The patient should be asked to sign the refusal form, and a family member, police officer, or bystander should sign as a witness to the patient's signing or witness the refusal to sign. The EMT should complete documentation of any assessment carried out and any refusal of the patient to assessment. The EMT should carefully document the conversation between the EMT and patient regarding refusal of care and consequences and should document the proposed care as well as the information the EMT gave the patient about alternate care (such as a visit to the personal physician) and the willingness to return if the patient has a change of mind.

Negligence

Negligence indicates that *proper care* has not been provided, based on established standards. *Reasonable care* uses a rationale for decision making in relation to providing care. State regulations regarding negligence may vary, but they all have some statutes of limitation, governmental immunity, and Good Samaritan laws that may provide a defense. Types of negligence include:

- Negligent conduct: Failure to provide reasonable care or to protect/assist another, based on existing standards and expertise.
- Gross negligence: Willfully providing inadequate care while disregarding safety/security.
- Contributory negligence: The injured party contributes to his/her own harm.
- Comparative negligence: The amount of negligence attributed to each individual involved.

If the charge of negligence is supported, the patient may collect physical (lost earnings due to injury), psychological (pain and suffering), and punitive damages.

Civil and Criminal Offenses

The four necessary elements of **negligence** (failure to follow the standards of care) are as follows:

1. Duty of care: The defendant (healthcare provider) had a duty to provide adequate care and/or protect the plaintiff's (patient's) safety.
2. Breach of duty: The defendant failed to carry out the duty to care, resulting in danger, injury, or harm to the plaintiff.
3. Damages: The plaintiff experienced illness or injury as a result of the breach of duty.
4. Causation: The plaintiff's illness or injury is directly caused by the defendant's negligent breach of duty.

Abandonment occurs if the EMT withdraws from providing care contrary to a patient's desire or knowledge and fails to arrange for appropriate care by others, resulting in harm to the patient. **Assault** occurs if an EMT threatens a patient in such a way that the patient becomes fearful of harm, whereas **battery** occurs when the EMT intentionally injures a patient, such as by hitting or shoving the person. Assault and battery often occur together.

Statutory Responsibilities and Mandatory Reporting

The EMT must practice within the **scope of responsibility**, which is outlined by each state's medical practice act. The EMT must be certified/licensed according to state requirements and meet appropriate educational standards regarding preparation and continuing education. The EMT has a duty to the patients, the medical director, and the public and functions under government and medical oversight.

Although laws about **mandatory reporting** vary from state to state, healthcare providers, including EMS personnel, are considered mandatory reporters in all states and must report suspected cases of child and elder abuse and neglect. The EMT must follow state guidelines for reporting because simply notifying the receiving facility of suspected abuse or neglect is not adequate. The EMT should be familiar with the signs of abuse and neglect (certain types of fractures; unexplained or multiple bruises; suspicious bruise patterns; burns; hair loss; and inadequate food, clothing, and shelter).

Evidence Preservation

When an incident may involve **court cases**, such as with gunshot wounds, knife, wounds, and rape, the EMT should take steps to **preserve evidence**, although providing emergent medical care takes priority. The EMT should try to avoid disturbing items at the scene of the incident and should assess the environment and document any unusual findings, remembering that the environment and the patient are both considered to be part of the crime scene. The EMT should collaborate with law enforcement officers at the scene. If the patient has had a gunshot wound or a knife wound, the EMT should not cut through the holes in the clothing but should cut along seams or away from the injuries. Any clothing or belongings removed during treatment should be secured separately in a paper bag (or plastic if paper is not available) and delivered with the patient to the receiving facility or to law enforcement officers. When the patient is describing the event, the EMT should document using quotations rather than summarizing.

Ethical Principles and Moral Obligations

Ethics is a branch of philosophy that studies morality—concepts of right and wrong. Applied ethics is the use of ethical principles, such as autonomy (right to self-determination), beneficence (acting to benefit another), nonmaleficence (doing no harm), verity (being truthful), and justice (equally distributing resources/care). Ethical conflicts may occur because of differences in cultural and ethical values, but they may also result from decisions that must be made regarding care, such as whether to provide CPR in a wilderness situation when the treatment is likely futile, situations involving triage in which some patients are given priority over others, situations that involve professional misconduct (such as EMS personnel being abusive toward patients), and incidents of patient dumping because the patient has inadequate insurance or an inability to pay. EMS personnel have a moral obligation to make decisions about care in good faith and in the patient's best interest.

Decision-Making Models

Do no harm	This model is based on nonmaleficence, the requirement that a treatment provided do no harm; however, by their nature, some treatments can and often do harm patients, so the underlying intent and goal of treatment must be considered when making decisions. For example, CPR may be carried out to save a patient's life and may be done with correct technique but still may result in rib fractures.
In good faith	The motive for a decision should be honest and fair, and decisions should be made with a sincere intention to do good even though the outcome may be negative. For example, EMS personnel may provide a treatment for a patient in good faith although the treatment proves to be ineffective for that particular patient.
Patient's best interest	Making a decision in the patient's best interest includes considering the patient's or parents' (in the case of children) wishes, the best clinical judgment, the best choice of various options, the chances for improvement/decline, and religious/cultural preferences.

Anatomy and Physiology

Body Planes and Anatomic Terms

Body planes include the following:

- Sagittal/Lateral: Vertical plane separating right from left.
- Median/Midsagittal: Sagittal plane at the midline (middle) separating the body into equal halves.
- Coronal/Frontal: Vertical plane separating anterior (front) from posterior (back).
- Axial/Transverse: Horizontal plane that separates the body into superior (upper) and inferior (lower) parts.
- A cross section is an axial/transverse (horizontal) cut through a tissue specimen or body structure, whereas a longitudinal section is a sagittal or coronal (vertical) cut.
- Medial is toward the midline, whereas lateral is away from the midline and to the side. Distal is farthest from the point of reference, and proximal is closest. When describing an area of the patient's body, the description should be patient oriented, using phrases such as "patient's left" and "patient's right" to ensure accurate interpretation.

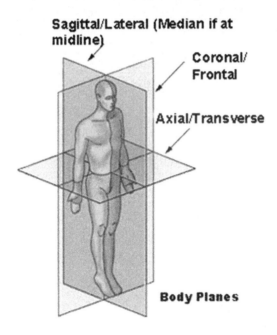

Sagittal/Lateral (Median if at midline)

Coronal/Frontal

Axial/Transverse

Body Planes

- 37 -

Medical Terminology

Common Medical Prefixes

Term	Meaning	Examples
Cardio-	Heart	Cardiovascular (heart and vessels), cardiology (study of the heart)
Neuro-	Nerves	Neurology (study of the nerves), neuron (nerve cell)
Hyper-	Enlarged, excessive, high	Hypertrophy (enlarged tissue), hyperemesis (excessive vomiting), hyperactive (overactive), hypertension (high BP)
Hypo-	Under, beneath, low	Hypoglycemia (low blood sugar), hypotension (low BP), hypoxia (low oxygen)
Naso-	Nose	Nasopharyngeal (nose and throat), nasal (referring to the nose)
Oro-	Mouth	Oropharyngeal (mouth and throat), oral (referring to the mouth)
Arterio-	Artery	Arteriovenous (artery and vein), arterial (referring to arteries)
Hemo- **Hemato-**	Blood	Hemolysis (breakdown of blood), hemoglobin (blood component), hematology (study of blood)
Therm-	Temperature	Thermoregulation (temperature regulation), thermometer (temperature measurement)
Vaso-	Vessels	Vasoconstriction (narrowing of vessels), vasodilation (widening of vessels)
Tachy-	Rapid	Tachycardia (rapid heart rate), tachypnea (rapid respirations)
Brady-	Slow	Bradycardia (slow heart rate), bradypnea (slow respirations)

Pathophysiology

Respiratory Compromise

Respiratory compromise may relate to problems with the following:

- Airway: The airway is blocked because of a foreign body, the tongue (especially in unconscious patients and young children), blood or secretions, edema (swelling), or trauma (blunt or penetrating).
- Respirations: The patient is unable to adequately breathe in enough oxygen because of inadequate oxygen in the environment, poison gases (such as carbon monoxide), lung infection (pneumonia), illness that narrows the breathing passages (chronic obstructive pulmonary disease [COPD], bronchitis), excess fluid in the lungs (pulmonary edema), excess fluid between the lung tissue and the blood vessels (leaving inadequate blood volume), and impaired circulation.
- Ventilation: The rate or depth of breathing is inadequate for air exchange; the volume of air breathed in is too small; or air exchange is impaired by altered consciousness, unconsciousness, chest injury, overdose of medication (such as narcotics), poisoning, and disease (such as amyotrophic lateral sclerosis [ALS], sometimes called Lou Gehrig's disease).

Shock

Shock, which is impaired blood flow to the body tissues (cells and organs), may relate to problems with the following:

- Heart: If the heart rate is too slow or too rapid and contractions are ineffectual, insufficient blood is pumped to the lungs for oxygenation and to the cells and body organs. Heart problems may relate to heart disease (such as heart failure), poisoning, and artificial ventilation that is excessive or ineffective.
- Blood vessels: Blood vessels may be unable to constrict, resulting in vasodilation and lowering of the BP. This most often occurs because of cervical (neck) spinal cord injuries, severe infection, or anaphylactic reaction.
- Blood: The volume of circulating blood or blood components may be inadequate to nurture the body cells and organs because of excessive bleeding or vomiting, diarrhea, or burns, which may result in dehydration.

Control of Respirations

The brain's **respiratory center** in the medulla oblongata responds to the body's chemical and mechanical signals. The medulla oblongata contains chemoreceptors that respond to changes in the pH in the fluid surrounding it and the carotid arteries and aorta contain peripheral chemoreceptors that respond to decreases in oxygen and pH. If the blood becomes more acidotic, the medulla oblongata increases the respiratory rate and the tidal volume. If the blood becomes more alkalotic, the medulla oblongata does the opposite in order to maintain the blood pH within the normal range. Mechanical/Stretch receptors are located in the lungs, upper airways, chest wall, and diaphragm, helping to control respirations. The stretch receptors respond when the lungs inflate and send a message to the medulla oblongata via the vagus nerve to prevent overinflation and vice versa. In healthy individuals, increases in carbon dioxide or a decrease in pH cause an increase in

- 39 -

the respiratory rate whereas increased oxygen decreases the respiratory rate. In conditions such as COPD in which carbon dioxide is chronically high, this mechanism is impaired.

Ventilation (V)/Perfusion (Q) Ratio and Mismatch

Ventilation (V) and perfusion (Q) are expressed in the ventilation/perfusion ratio (V/Q ratio). Ideally, the volume of blood perfusing the lungs (4–5 L) should equal the volume of gas reaching the alveoli each minute throughout all parts of the lungs, providing a V/Q ratio of 1:1. However, V and Q do not always match, a situation referred to as V/Q mismatch. For example, there is more ventilation than perfusion at the lung apices and less ventilation than perfusion at the lung bases. Additionally, some diseases and conditions may cause V/Q mismatch, such as COPD, severe asthma, pneumonia, pulmonary embolism, and atelectasis. Ventilation may be limited (such as with asthma) while perfusion remains stable, resulting in hypoxemia because of an inadequate intake of oxygen. A pulmonary embolus or other disease may block an area of the lung so that ventilation is adequate but perfusion is impaired, again resulting in hypoxemia.

Myocardial Effectiveness

Myocardial effectiveness depends on cardiac output, the volume of blood pumped from the left ventricle of the heart in one minute, and it equals the stroke volume (the volume of blood ejected with each ventricular contraction, usually about 70 mL in an adult) times the heart rate. So, if the heart rate is 60, the cardiac output (60 × 70) would be 4200 mL (normally 4–8 L/min). <u>Stroke volume</u> is determined by the following factors:

- <u>Preload</u>: Stretch/Tension of muscle fibers, usually corresponding to the end-diastolic pressure when the ventricles are filled.
- <u>Afterload</u>: The amount of pressure that the ventricles must work against when ejecting blood during systole, representing the systemic vascular resistance.
- <u>Myocardial contractility:</u> The amount of stretch in the myocardial muscle fibers, which determines the forcefulness of the contractions.

Systemic vascular resistance increases when vessels constrict and decreases when they dilate. With atherosclerosis, the vessels become more rigid and the lumen (opening) tends to narrow from plaque deposits, increasing systemic vascular resistance and increasing the burden on the heart.

Blood Pressure (BP)

Blood pressure (BP; the force of the blood against the vessel walls) is necessary to maintain adequate perfusion. BP relates to cardiac output (CO) and systemic vascular resistance (SVR) (aka total peripheral resistance). SVR results from the resistance of the blood flow from the lumen (opening) of the vessel and the viscosity of the blood. The mechanisms that control BP affect either the CO or the SVR. If the CO remains stable but the SVR increases, then the BP rises. Although the stroke volume often varies little, the heart rate can increase markedly, affecting cardiac output. As the CO increases, the BP increases. If the CO decreases, then the BP decreases as well. As the SVR increases, the BP increases; and as the SVR decreases, the BP decreases. The body responds to changes in CO, SVR, and BP through vasoconstriction, which increases the SVR and BP, and vasodilation, which decreases the SVR and BP. Thus, if a patient is in shock and the CO and BP fall, the body reacts with vasoconstriction to increase the BP.

Life Span Development

Normal Vital Signs from Neonate to Older Adulthood

Age	Heart rate	Respirations	BP (mm Hg)
Neonate (newborn)	100–220 (average 140–160) begins to slow after 3 months	40–60 for a few minutes, then 30–40	Systolic 70–90
Toddler (12–36 mos.)	80–130	20–30	Systolic 70–100
Preschool (3 to 5)	80–120	20–30	Systolic 80–110
School age (6-12)	70–110	20–30	80–120/60–80
Adolescence (13–18)	55–100	12–20	110–131/64–84
Early adulthood (19–40)	60–100 (average 80)	12–20	100–119/60–79 to 140/90 (high)
Middle adulthood (41–60)	60–100 (average 80)	12–20	100–119/60–79 to 140/90 (high)
Late adulthood (61+)	60–100 (average 70)	12–20	100–119/60–79 to 140/90 (high)

Levels of Disease Prevention

Levels of disease prevention include the following:

- Primary: The goal is to prevent the initial occurrence of a health problem, such as a disease or injury, through activities such as immunizations, smoking cessation, fluoride supplementation of water, promotion of seat belt and helmet use, and use of child car seat restraints. Interventions are often aimed at the general public or large groups of people.
- Secondary: The goal is to identify diseases or conditions quickly and provide prompt intervention to provide treatment and prevent further disability through activities such as BP screenings, breast and testicular self-examinations, hearing and vision screenings, mammography, and pregnancy testing.
- Tertiary: The goal is to assist those who already have disease or disability to prevent further progress of the disease and to allow people to achieve the maximum quality of life through activities such as support groups, counseling, diet and exercise, stress management, and supportive services.

Public Health

Public Health System

EMS are part of the **public health system**, a network of private, nonprofit, and government agencies and healthcare providers providing public health services in a wide range of areas. The primary services provided by the public health system include the following:

- Monitoring community health.
- Identifying hazards to health in the environment/community.
- Educating people about health issues.
- Mobilizing various agencies and individuals to take action.
- Enforcing public safety laws/regulations.
- Ensuring that healthcare providers are qualified, licensed, and certified as required.
- Ensuring that health care is available.
- Assessing the effectiveness of health care.
- Researching health problems and finding solutions.

Public health laws/regulations may be federal, state, or tribal and cover issues such as immunization requirements, drinking water/sewage system standards, air quality, water fluoridation, restrictions on tobacco use (age and place), restrictions on drinking (age, driving), speed limits, prenatal care, abuse (child, older adult, sexual, and domestic), safety equipment, and safe lifting. Healthy People 2020, of the U.S. Department of Health and Human Services, provides goals and objectives for health-related public policies.

Safety Equipment and Education

Safety equipment may include a wide variety of devices, including smoke alarms and carbon monoxide alarms. Some safety equipment protects people from falls, especially older adults. These may include safety rails, grab bars, canes, and walkers. EMS personnel are often involved in public education regarding the following:

- <u>Car seats:</u> Should be properly secured in the backseat of a motor vehicle. They should be rear facing for infants and toddlers up to 2 years of age (or the maximum recommended height and weight) and forward-facing with a harness for toddlers and preschoolers. School-aged children should use booster seats with a belt and harness until they are at least 4 feet 9 inches tall. Children younger than age 13 should not ride in a front seat.
- <u>Seat belts:</u> All people in a motor vehicle should be secured with seat belts and shoulder harnesses.
- <u>Helmets:</u> Should fit properly and snugly, cover the top of the forehead, and have a securing chinstrap. They should be worn when riding a bicycle or motorcycle and engaging in sports activities such as rollerblading but not on playground equipment or when climbing trees.

Pharmacology

Pharmacodynamics and Pharmacokinetics

Pharmacodynamics relates to biological effects (therapeutic or adverse) of drug administration. Responses may be continuous, such as BP variations, or dichotomous, in which an event either occurs or does not (such as recovery). Information from pharmacodynamics provides feedback to modify medication dosage (pharmacokinetics). **Pharmacokinetics** relates to the route of administration, the absorption, the dosage, the frequency of administration, the distribution, and the serum levels achieved over time. Most drugs are cleared through the kidneys. Elimination half-time is the time needed to reduce plasma concentrations to 50% during elimination. Age and weight may impact the absorption and elimination of drugs. Drugs have a generic/scientific/nonproprietary name (acetaminophen) and a brand/trade/proprietary name (Tylenol). Emergency medications include solids (pills, capsules, powders), liquids (enteral [ingested] or parenteral [injected]), and gases (inhaled). Enteral medications may be given orally (glucose) or sublingually (nitroglycerin). Parenteral drugs are inhaled (oxygen, albuterol) or injected (epinephrine).

Commonly Administered Medications

Medication	Dose/Route/Use	Side effects/Interactions
Aspirin	Orally, 325 mg, chew and swallow for fast action when having a heart attack.	Avoid with signs of stroke or gastrointestinal (GI) bleeding. Decreases clotting time and may increase the risk of bleeding.
Glucose	Orally for hypoglycemia. May be in liquid or tablet form, or a glass of orange juice may be given.	Minimal unless hyperglycemic.
Oxygen	Inhaled, usually 2–6 L, but it varies according to protocol.	Minimal, although oxygen toxicity can occur with high doses for prolonged periods of time.
Bronchodilators (albuterol, levalbuterol)	Inhaled, usually two puffs of a handheld inhaler. Dosage varies according to the medication. For bronchospasm, wheezing.	Adverse effects: tachycardia, dizziness, nervousness, tremor, headache, rhinitis, increased cough.
Epinephrine (EpiPen)	Autoinjector, 0.3 mg 1:1000 for ≥66 lb. 0.15 mg 1:2000 for 33–66 lb. for severe allergic reaction/anaphylaxis.	Avoid using with antihistamines, thyroid hormones, and alpha blockers. Adverse effects: drowsiness, headache, palpitations, nervousness, tremors.
Nitroglycerin	Sublingually for angina (chest pain), 0.3–0.6 mg, repeated every 5 minutes up to three times.	Avoid with myocardial infarction. Adverse effects: headache, flushing, dizziness, orthostatic hypotension, palpitations. Interactions: Avoid with erectile dysfunction drugs (sildenafil, tadalafil, vardenafil).

Assistance with Medications and the Five Rights of Medication Administration

The EMT may assist patients to self-administer medications or administer them directly depending on the scope of practice and protocols. Medical direction may be offline, which means standing orders are available to treat specific conditions or written protocols have been established that must be followed. On-line medical direction requires verbal contact with a medical director. When receiving an on-line medication order, the EMT should use the echo technique (repeating back the orders to ensure that they were understood correctly) and clarify any orders that are confusing or unclear.

The **five rights of medication administration** include the following:

1. Right patient: The medication should be prescribed specifically for that patient.
2. Right medication: Correct choice for the patient's condition, and it matches the prescription.
3. Right route: Appropriate for the patient's condition, enteral or parenteral.
4. Right dose: As prescribed and appropriate for the patient's age, weight, and condition.
5. Right time: The medication is not expired, and it is administered at the time ordered, such as "stat" (immediately) or "every 5 minutes × 3."

Airway Management, Respirations and Artificial Ventilation

Respiratory (Airway) System

Air enters the **respiratory system** through the nose and mouth, where it is warmed and moistened, and it passes through the <u>pharynx</u> (back of throat) and the <u>larynx</u> (voice box) into the <u>trachea</u> (windpipe). The <u>epiglottis</u> is a cartilage flap that closes over the larynx when swallowing so food enters the esophagus (the tube leading to the stomach). The trachea branches into the right and left <u>bronchi</u> (large tubes) that carry the air into the <u>lungs</u>. Each bronchus branches into smaller <u>bronchioles</u> and millions of <u>alveoli</u> (small air sacs), which are covered with webs of tiny capillaries that deliver carbon dioxide and pick up oxygen (external respiration). The muscles of respiration are the <u>diaphragm</u> and the <u>intercostal muscles</u> (between the ribs), but <u>accessory muscles</u> in the neck and collarbone area may help during respiratory distress. The heart circulates unoxygenated blood to the lungs. After oxygenation, the blood returns to the heart and into the general circulation and body cells where gas exchange occurs again (internal respiration). Cells intake oxygen and nutrients and release carbon dioxide and waste products (cellular respiration).

Pediatrics: Infants are obligate nasal breathers for the first two to four months and usually only breathe through the nose, although they can generally breathe through the mouth if necessary. However, if nasal passages are blocked, they may quickly develop respiratory distress. Chest wall compliance is greater in infants and small children, so they must work harder than an adult to move the same amount of air. Additionally, proportionally the airway is smaller, the tongue is larger, and the cartilage is softer, increasing the risk of obstruction.

Older adults: Breathing capacity tends to decline after age 40 because the number of alveoli decreases and the size of alveoli increases, resulting in less surface for and less efficient gas exchange. Lung elasticity also decreases, resulting in decreased vital capacity. The chest muscles tend to weaken and stiffen with age, and older adults have a lowered ability to cough and clear the airways.

Life Support Chain

Critical to the **life support chain** are oxygenation and perfusion. Oxygenation involves gas exchange of carbon dioxide for oxygen at the alveolar/capillary level and the cell/capillary level. Perfusion involves the transport of blood, which carries oxygen, glucose, and other nutrients as well as waste products throughout the body. Oxygen and glucose are essential for cell functioning. Glucose is produced by the digestion of carbohydrates (starches); it is the primary energy source for the body; and its use is controlled by insulin, which is produced by the pancreas. Excess glucose is stored in the liver as glycogen for later use or is converted to fat. These fundamental elements are affected by the composition of ambient air (usually 21% oxygen), airway patency, ventilation, regulation of respiration, blood volume and transport, heart action, and blood vessel size and resistance.

Terms Associated with the Physiology of Respiration

Tidal volume	Normal volume of gas inhaled during one respiration cycle (approximately 500 mL in a healthy adult).
Inspiratory reserve volume	Volume of air inhaled greater than the tidal volume during forced deep inhalation (up to 3000 mL).
Dead space	Volume of inhaled gas that does not take part in gas exchange.
Alveolar dead space	Volume of alveoli that are ventilated but not perfused.
Vital capacity	Maximum volume of gas that can be forcefully exhaled from the lungs following a full inhalation.
Minute volume	Volume of gas expelled from the lungs in one minute (the respiratory rate × the tidal volume).
Residual volume	Volume of gas remaining in the lungs after one full, forced exhalation.
Total lung capacity	Vital capacity plus residual volume; it is the total volume that the lungs can contain (usually about 6000 mL for adults).
Cellular respiration	Use of oxygen and glucose to produce energy at the cellular level and the creation of water and carbon dioxide as by-products of metabolism.
Oxygenation	Process by which oxygen molecules bind to hemoglobin in the blood.

Airway Assessment and Manual Measures to Clear the Airway

Indications of an adequate airway include a normal voice and speaking ability and audible and visible air exchange. Indications of inadequate airway include unusual breathing sounds (wheezing, stridor), hoarse voice/inability to speak, and no audible or visible air exchange. Airway obstruction may result from the tongue falling back, food, a foreign body, vomit, blood, teeth, and edema (swelling). **Maneuvers** include the following:

- Head tilt/chin lift: Hyperextend the neck by tilting the patient's head back with one hand on his or her forehead to straighten the airway and lift the tongue. Then lift the chin and pull forward with the fingers of the other hand under the chin with the thumb on top. The chin lift pulls the mandible (jaw) forward. This prevents the tongue from blocking the pharynx. Contraindications to the head tilt/chin lift include suspected cervical spine and neck injuries.
- Jaw thrust: This technique is used with a suspected spinal cord or neck injury in which extending the neck must be avoided. From behind, place the fingers behind the angles of the patient's lower jaw and place your thumbs on the chin; move the jaw upward until it is extended while using the thumbs to slightly open the patient's mouth. Contraindications include severe facial injuries.
- Modified chin lift/jaw thrust: This technique is used with a suspected spinal cord/neck injury with an unstable cervical spine. From the head of the patient, place your thumbs on his or her cheekbones and place your fingers under the patient's mandible, and then pull the mandible upward with the fingers while applying pressure with the thumbs. If using a mask for ventilation, place the mask in position and secure it with your thumbs while your fingers thrust the patient's jaw forward.

Ventilation

Ventilation is adequate if the respiratory rate, depth of respiration, and effort of breathing are normal. Signs of inadequate ventilation include the following:

- Increased effort of breathing: Nasal flaring, sternal retraction (infants), use of abdominal or intercostal (between the ribs) muscles, sweating, sitting in the tripod position (upright, leaning forward, hands on knees).
- Abnormal breath sounds: Wheezes, rales (crackles), and/or rhonchi (snoring/whistling sounds).
- Abnormal depth of breathing: Hypoventilation (too shallow) or hyperventilation (too deep).
- Abnormal rate of breathing: Tachypnea (too fast) or bradypnea (too slow).
- Abnormal chest wall movement: Splinting, asymmetric, paradoxical (chest wall/diaphragm move in during inhalation and out during exhalation—opposite of normal).
- Irregular breathing pattern: May include periods of apnea (no breathing).

Patients with inadequate ventilation or apnea in which there is no breathing or only occasional gasping require ventilation assistance, such as with a pocket mask or bag-valve mask (BVM).

Oropharyngeal Airway (OPA)

The **oropharyngeal airway** (OPA), a blind-insertion airway device, may be inserted to provide better ventilation, but the OPA requires the head tilt/chin lift or modified jaw thrust as well because the device alone does not ensure a patent airway. The OPA is indicated for unconscious patients, patients with no gag reflex, and patients who are apneic (not breathing) and require ventilatory aid. The OPA is often inserted if a patient stops breathing, such as with a cardiac arrest. The OPA is contraindicated in conscious patients and those with a gag reflex. To insert the OPA, perform the following steps:

- Estimate the length of the OPA by measuring the patient from the angle of the jaw or the tip of the earlobe to the corner of the mouth.
- Select the correct size.
- Open the patient's mouth using the cross-finger technique. Suction any secretions.
- Tilt the head back (if possible). Insert the device with the tip of the OPA pointing upward for adults and downward for children.
- Rotate the OPA into position for adults.
- Ensure that the phalanges of the mouthpiece are securely against the patient's mouth.
- Check to make sure the OPA is patent (open).

Nasopharyngeal Airway (NPA)

The **nasopharyngeal airway** (NPA), a blind-insertion airway device, is indicated for unconscious or semiconscious patients who still have a gag reflex or those who cannot tolerate an oropharyngeal airway (OPA), but it should be avoided with severe head injury, risk of basal skull fracture, nasal bleeding, and history of deviated septum or nasal fracture. It's important to use the appropriate size. To insert the NPA, perform the following steps: Choose a size that is slightly smaller in diameter than the patient's nostril. Measure from the tip of the earlobe to the tip of the nose. Lubricate the NPA with water-soluble lubricant and insert it in the larger and most patent (open) nostril. If inserting into the right nostril, insert with the bevel (tip) angled toward the nasal septum (the bony cartilage division between the nostrils). If inserting it into the left nostril, invert the NPA to angle the bevel toward the septum. When the NPA reaches the throat, rotate it 180° into the proper position.

Bag-Valve Mask (BVM)

Bag-valve mask (BVM) ventilation equipment used for positive-pressure ventilation (PPV) includes a mask, a ventilator bag, an oxygen reservoir bag, and an attachment for oxygen delivery. The correct mask size is important: The mask should not cover the chin. BVM is contraindicated if the airway is not patent, but it is used for abnormal breathing and for respiratory distress/failure. BVM requires two EMS personnel—one to control the mask and the other to control the bag. Steps are as follows:

- Position yourself behind the patient's head, place the mask over the patient's nose and mouth, and make a tight seal by holding it in place with your thumbs and index fingers while your other fingers slide under the patient's jaw to lift the chin.
- Squeeze the bag with inhalations initially for 5 to 10 breaths and then adjust the rate to at least 12 breaths per minute, slowly adjusting the rate and tidal volume delivered.

Assessment of lung compliance (the ability to expand and contract) includes observation of chest movement, rate of respirations, and the feel of BVM. Difficult ventilation suggests impaired compliance. Note: The BVM can be used with or without oxygen.

Sellick's Maneuver (Cricoid Pressure)

Sellick's maneuver (cricoid pressure) may be used with PPV to prevent air from flowing down the esophagus and into the stomach rather than down the trachea and into the lungs because stomach distension increases the risk of vomiting. This maneuver may also be used with intubation to prevent regurgitation of stomach contents and aspiration. Sellick's maneuver may be used on unconscious patients receiving a mask or BVM. The procedure consists of applying pressure downward to the cricoid cartilage of the neck (which is at the bottom of the larynx and blocks the upper esophagus) with the thumb and index finger. Pressure is usually applied at 30 to 40 newtons but no greater than 40 newtons because too great of force may block the airway. The maneuver may also cause nausea and vomiting and, with severe pressure, may result in rupture of the esophagus. Vomiting is a contraindication.

Normal Negative-Pressure Breathing and Positive-Pressure Breathing

Negative-pressure breathing (normal)	Positive-pressure breathing
The movement downward of the diaphragm (triggered by the phrenic nerves) creates a negative pressure in the lungs, drawing air into them.	Ventilation forces air into the lungs, and this can result in dysfunction of the diaphragm because it is responding to a change in pressure rather than stimulation by the phrenic nerve.
Blood flows from the lungs to the heart and back and to the body at a steady rate in normal breathing.	Blood flow from the lungs is reduced, resulting in decreased cardiac (heart) output.
The epiglottis closes the esophagus during inhalation, preventing air from entering the stomach.	The epiglottis may stay open during ventilation, allowing air into the stomach and increasing the risk of vomiting.

Recovery Position

The **recovery position** is used for patients who are unconscious but breathing (such as those with a drug overdose or after a seizure) and have no life-threatening injuries. This position helps to maintain a patent airway and reduces the risk of aspiration from vomitus.

	Kneeling beside the patient, lift his or her chin to ensure that the airway is open and place his or her closest arm at right angle to body with hand up. Place the patient's farthest arm around his or her neck with the hand touching the opposite cheek. Flex the patient's knee to 90° until the foot is flat on the floor/surface.
	Using the patient's knee as a fulcrum and supporting the farthest arm and shoulder, roll the patient onto his or her side by pulling on the farthest knee. Make sure that the top knee contacts the floor/surface to support the patient's body and that the top hand is under his or her head to keep the neck in a neutral position.

Upper Airway Suctioning

Suctioning devices may be vehicle mounted or portable and should be checked to ensure that the tubing is intact and the canister has an airtight seal. Patients at risk for aspiration include those with an altered level of consciousness, those having difficulty swallowing or breathing, trauma patients, obese patients, and those with recurrent vomiting. Oral suctioning is used to remove secretions, vomitus, and blood. Suctioning may be done with a rigid-tip catheter (Yankauer) or a soft-tip catheter. Techniques include the following:

- Don a mask and gloves.
- Measure the patient from the tip of the ear to the corner of the mouth to determine how far to insert the catheter.
- Turn on the suction.
- Use the cross-finger technique to open the mouth.
- Insert the tube and apply suction. The rigid catheter has a finger control to start and stop suction.
- Move the catheter around the gum line and over the tongue to the back of the mouth, but avoid stimulating the gag reflex.
- Suction for no longer than 15 seconds at a time.
- Note: Clear a small infant's airway by suctioning the nose with a bulb syringe.

Portable Oxygen Cylinders

Two commonly used sizes of **portable oxygen cylinders** are D tanks (M15; 350 L) and E tanks (M24; 625 L). The EMT should use protective equipment (goggles, gloves). The cylinder should be placed upright. A label over the holes on the top of the cylinder indicates that the cylinder is full. Remove the label, leaving the washers in place unless the washers are built into the regulator. Face the opening of the tank away, and use the key to crack the cylinder by letting out a small amount of oxygen. Apply the regulator and slide it into place. Tighten and then open the cylinder to check for pressure (there should be at least 200 psi). Close the cylinder, attach the oxygen tubing to the regulator, set the oxygen flow to the correct amount of liters, and then open the cylinder and

- 49 -

administer oxygen to the patient. When discontinuing use of the cylinder, turn off the cylinder, remove the oxygen tubing, turn the oxygen flow setting up to bleed air from the regular, and remove the regulator.

Physiology of Respiration

The **physiology of respiration** includes the following:

- Ventilation: Movement of air in and out of the lungs during inhalation and exhalation. The normal tidal volume (air exchange when breathing normally) for an adult is about 500 mL, but it is lower for infants and children (5–7 mL/kg for neonates, 6–8 mL/kg for children). Breathing may be impaired by disease (muscular dystrophy), drugs, trauma, bronchoconstriction, allergic reactions, foreign body obstructions, and infection.
- Oxygenation: The process by which oxygen molecules bind to hemoglobin in the blood. The blood saturation level reflects the amount of oxygen that is dissolved in the blood and available to body tissues, and it should be ≥95%.
- Respiration: The process by which the lungs exchange carbon dioxide for oxygen in the alveoli and provide this oxygenated blood to body tissues. Respiration may be external (inspiration, expiration), internal (exchange of gas), or cellular (cells perform tasks that require oxygen and glucose [sugar] and produce carbon dioxide as a waste product). Respiration may be impaired by a lack of air, toxins/poisons, and ineffective circulation (shock, cardiac arrest).

Assessment of Oxygenation

Assessment of oxygenation includes the following:

- Evaluate respirations: Note the signs of respiratory distress—rapid breathing, slow breathing, use of accessory muscles, nasal flaring, and sternal retraction—because they may indicate inadequate oxygenation.
- Assess mental status: Confusion may be associated with hypo-oxygenation (low oxygen), but it's important to determine a baseline mental status if possible because the patient may have dementia or may be confused because of medications.
- Assess skin: Note cyanosis (blue tinge) especially around the mouth, fingertips, and oral mucous membranes because this indicates a lack of oxygen. Another sign is pallor. Mottling of the skin, purplish or reddish discoloration especially on the knees and feet, indicates hypo-oxygenation and is a common indication that death is near.
- Monitor pulse oximetry: It should be 95%–100%. If a patient has mild respiratory disease, the pulse oximetry level may be as low as 90% and still be within the normal range for the patient. Readings less than 90%–92% indicate hypoxemia (low oxygen in the blood).

Assessment of Respirations and Supplemental Oxygen Administration

When **assessing respirations**, the EMT should note the patient's gag reflex and rate of respirations (whether it is normal for the patient's age or it is too fast, too slow, or absent). The EMT should also evaluate the rise and fall of the chest and any abnormal movements (such as sternal retraction, nasal flaring) noisy breathing (gurgling, wheezing), the use of accessory muscles, or the tripod position (sitting, leaning forward, and supporting the body with the hands). If breathing is abnormal or the pulse oximetry is less than 95%, the EMT should take precautions against bloodstream infection (BSI) and administer **supplemental oxygen** with a nonrebreather mask with the oxygen set at 12–15 L. The reservoir bag of the mask must be completely filled before applying the mask to the patient, securing it with an elastic band about the head. If the patient cannot tolerate the nonrebreather mask, then a <u>nasal cannula</u> may be used with the oxygen flow set at 4–6 L, the prongs inserted into the nostrils, and tubing secured by looping over the ears and tightening under the chin.

Pulse Oximetry

Pulse oximetry uses an external oximeter that attaches to the patient's finger or earlobe to measure arterial oxygen saturation (SPO_2), the percentage of hemoglobin that is saturated with oxygen. The oximeter uses light waves to determine SPO_2. Oxygen saturation should be maintained >95%, although some patients with chronic respiratory disorders, such as COPD, may have lower SPO_2 readings. Results may be compromised by impaired circulation, excessive light, poor positioning, and nail polish. If the SPO_2 reading falls, the oximeter should be repositioned because incorrect positioning is a common cause of inaccurate readings. Oximetry is used for monitoring when patients are on oxygen or mechanical ventilation. Oximeters do not provide information about carbon dioxide levels, so they cannot monitor carbon dioxide retention. Oximeters also cannot differentiate between different forms of hemoglobin, so if the hemoglobin has picked up carbon monoxide, the oximeter will not recognize that.

Oxygen Delivery Devices

Oxygen delivery devices provide oxygen-enriched air. Ambient air is about 21% oxygen, so the fraction of inspired air (FIO_2) is 21%.

Oxygen delivery devices	
Nasal cannula (prongs)	FIO_2 of 24%–40% with flows of ≤6 liters per minute (LPM). Humidification should be used for prolonged flow rates of >4 LPM.
Partial rebreather face mask	This mask covers the nose and mouth, delivering FIO_2 of 30%–60%, but the flow of oxygen should be maintained between 6 and 12 LPM to decrease the risk of rebreathing. Because of the higher flow rate, humidification should be used.
Venturi mask	Oxygen entrainment masks come with different-sized color-coded nozzles to more accurately control FIO_2, with different sizes providing different FIO_2 levels, usually ranging from 24% to 50%, although an FIO_2 reading of >35% is not always reliable. The flow rate is 12–15 LPM. Humidifiers may be used.
Non-rebreather mask	This mask covers the mouth and nose with a reservoir bag of oxygen. A one-way valve prevents the patient from rebreathing exhaled air. FIO_2 is about 60%–80% or greater at a flow rate of 15 LPM.

Positive Airway Pressure (PAP) Devices

All **positive airway pressure** (PAP) devices, such as <u>continuous positive airway pressure</u> (CPAP), have an air blower that delivers pressurized room air to an interface/mask. Pressure can be increased or decreased by adjusting the speed or the amount of airflow, with most machines generating from 2 to 20 cm of water pressure. Carbon dioxide is expelled through a vent or a nonrebreather valve on expiration. <u>Bilevel PAP (BiPAP, BPAP)</u> devices deliver two levels of pressure, which can be preset. Inspiratory PAP (IPAP) is set at a higher level (10 cm H_2O) than is expiratory PAP (EPAP) (5 cm H_2O) to allow a higher pressure needed to open the airway during inspiration but reduce the pressure to facilitate expiration. PAP is indicated for pulmonary edema, CHF, COPD, asthma, and near drowning.

The procedure includes the following:

- Fill the humidifier with distilled water.
- Program the settings.
- Fit the mask and headgear/straps.
- Begin with the pressure at the lowest setting, usually 5 cm H_2O (CPAP), and increase it slowly at 1 cm H_2O every few minutes until the optimal level is reached.
- Monitor the oxygen saturation and respirations.

Pocket-Mask Ventilation

Pocket-mask ventilation is used when administering cardiopulmonary resuscitation (CPR) to a patient who is in cardiac arrest and apneic (not breathing). If two EMS personnel are available, one should be positioned at the patient's head to administer pocket-mask ventilation while the other does compressions. If there is only one EMS personnel, then that person should be positioned at the patient's side. Administration is as follows:

- Remove the mask from the container and push the flattened mask to open it.
- Wipe the patient's face clean with alcohol swab if necessary to remove secretions, vomitus.
- Do a chin tilt or jaw thrust and place the mask over the patient's nose and mouth, holding it in place with both hands to seal it tightly.
- Take a deep breath and blow in through the one-way valve, watching the chest rise to ensure that ventilation has occurred.
- Continue to ventilate the patient at a rate of 30 compressions to 2 ventilations for CPR.
- Attach supplemental oxygen if available to improve oxygenation.
- Upon patient recovery or completion of CPR, remove the mask, discard the valve, and disinfect the mask.

Positive End-Expiratory Pressure (PEEP)

Positive end-expiratory pressure (PEEP) is a setting in mechanical ventilation, that is, the airway pressure at the end of an exhalation. The primary purpose of PEEP is to improve oxygenation by preventing airway collapse. The usual settings are 5 to 25 cm H_2O. PEEP is indicated for respiratory distress syndromes/acute lung injury, pulmonary edema, atelectasis, and severe pneumonia resulting in hypoxemia. PEEP may improve gas exchange and lung compliance and prevent alveolar collapse, but it may also decrease gas exchange and cardiac output and cause hypotension and hypoperfusion of internal organs as well as barotrauma and increased intracranial pressure. PEEP is contraindicated with increased intracranial pressure, low cardiac output, pneumothorax (without a pleural catheter), and hypovolemia. The procedure is as follows:

Start the setting at 5 cm H_2O, and increase it by 2–3 cm H_2O (not to exceed 15) every 30 to 60 minutes to achieve oxygen saturation of greater than 88% or PaO_2 of greater than 55 mm Hg.

Assessment

Primary Assessment

After surveying the environment for safety issues, the EMT should quickly conduct a **primary assessment** to identify conditions that are life-threatening, as follows:

- Level of consciousness: Alert, responsive to verbal stimuli, responsive to painful stimuli, nonresponsive.
- Breathing status: Normal, abnormal, rate abnormalities (>24 or <8), apnea, choking, normal or abnormal chest movement, chest rise and fall, noisy respirations, use of accessory muscles, tripod position, nasal flaring.
- Circulatory status: Radial, carotid pulse, pulse abnormalities, major bleeding, skin color—pink, blue (cyanotic), pale, skin temperature, skin moisture, capillary refill, signs of shock.

Life-threatening conditions must be treated immediately, as follows:

- If there is no radial pulse but there is a carotid pulse, lie the patient flat and elevate his or her feet 8 to 12 inches.
- No pulse: Begin CPR.
- Shock: Lay the patient flat, elevate his or her feet 8–12 inches, and administer oxygen at 15 L/min.
- Bleeding: Apply pressure to control any bleeding.
- Abnormal breathing: Provide oxygen with a nonrebreather mask. If the patient is unresponsive, cyanotic, or in respiratory distress, use a BVM with supplemental oxygen.
- Unresponsive: Ensure a patent airway.

Based on the assessment, the patient is classified as stable, potentially unstable, or unstable.

History Taking on Arrival at a Scene

History taking should include the following:

- <u>Chief complaint:</u> If the patient is unable to explain, information may be gathered from his or her family, friends, or others who are present. Look for a medical alert bracelet or other such jewelry.
- <u>Nature of the illness or mechanism of injury:</u> Reason for calling EMS, cause of injury, type of illness. Look for environmental clues (fire, drug paraphernalia, motor vehicle accident).
- <u>Signs and symptoms observed or reported by the patient:</u> Skin temperature, open wounds, BP abnormalities, pain, or difficulty breathing.
- <u>Precipitating events:</u> Falls, accidents, violence, eating, exercising, walking, driving.
- <u>Pediatric considerations:</u> Check capillary refill to assess blood flow in infants and children younger than 6. Assess the pulse at the brachial artery (inside of the upper arm) for infants up to 1 year of age and the carotid artery in the neck for children older than 1 year. May need to use distraction to gain trust and alleviate fear. Encourage the parents/caregivers to hold <u>the </u>child if possible and assist in calming the child.
- <u>Geriatric (older adult) considerations:</u> Determine if the patient needs assistive devices, such as hearing aids, eyeglasses, cane, walker, or dentures.

OPQRST Method of History Taking

O	Onset	The time that the symptoms associated with this event started.
P	Provocative; palliative. Positioning	That which makes it better; that which makes it worse. The position that the patient is in on arrival and the need to remain in this position or to move him or her.
Q	Quality of discomfort	Burning, stabbing, nagging, crushing, sharp, or dull.
R	Radiation of pain	Area to which the pain moves from the original site.
S	Severity of pain	Based on a 1-to-10 or other appropriate scale.
T	Time	Historical onset, such as earlier, similar events.

SAMPLE Method of History Taking

S	Signs and symptoms	Pain, bleeding, shortness of breath, injuries, fever, rash.
A	Allergies	Medications, environmental (foods, insects, plants, animals).
M	Medications	Prescribed, over-the-counter (OTC) vitamins/minerals, birth control and erectile dysfunction medications, herbal preparations, recreational drugs, other people's medications.
P	Past pertinent history	Especially related to the current event.
L	Last oral intake	Foods, fluids, other substances.
E	Events (precipitating)	Occurrence just prior to event.

Taking a History of Sensitive Topics

When asking a patient about **sensitive topics,** the EMT should try to provide as much privacy as possible in an emergent situation in order to maintain confidentiality and protect the patient from reprisals. The EMT should ask questions directly in a straightforward and nonjudgmental manner, stressing the need for information in order to help the patient, especially if the patient is reluctant to answer. Sensitive topics include the following:

- Sexual history: People who engage in unusual or unhealthy sexual practices, such as sadomasochism, autoerotic asphyxiation, swinging, and prostitution, are often reluctant to admit to those practices. Adolescents may be especially reluctant to admit they are pregnant or have engaged in sexual activity or have had an abortion. Males (especially those older than age 40) should be asked about the use of erectile dysfunction drugs (such as Viagra) because they are a contraindication to some medical treatments.
- Physical/Sexual abuse and/or violence: Victims often lie about abuse to defend the abuser or out of shame or fear of further violence.
- Alcohol/Drug use and abuse: Patients often underreport the extent of their drinking or drug taking or deny it altogether. Patients may be concerned about legal actions, such as if they have been driving drunk and gotten into an accident.

Special History-Taking Challenges

Special history-taking challenges include the following:

- Silent patient: Be patient, sensitive, and alert for nonverbal clues.
- Talkative patient: Allow the patient to speak freely for a few minutes and then periodically summarize.
- Anxious patient: Be patient, provide reassurance, and explain all procedures.
- Patient with multiple complaints: Ask the patient to help prioritize his or her issues.
- Hostile/angry patient: Remain calm; respond as appropriate.
- Intoxicated patient: Avoid cornering, belittling, or challenging the patient or asking the patient to lower his or her voice or stop swearing. Remain calm and treat the patient with respect.
- Depressed, crying patient: Question the severity of the patient's depression; listen and remain supportive and nonjudgmental.
- Patient with a language barrier: Use a translator if possible. Use hand gestures. Show the equipment before using it; point to the part of the body where the equipment will be used.
- Patient with a visual impairment: Announce your presence and explain all procedures verbally. Tell the patient before touching him or her.
- Patient with a hearing impairment: Determine if the patient has a hearing aid, and obtain it if possible. Speak slowly and clearly, facing the patient for any hearing deficit. If the patient has no hearing, use writing, hand gestures, and demonstrations to communicate.

Secondary Assessment

Following completion of the primary assessment and after attending to any life-threatening problems that are identified, carry out **a secondary assessment** as follows:

- Measure vital signs: Pulse (radial to carotid for adults and brachial for infants and small children), respiration rate, and BP. Using the correct BP cuff size is essential for accuracy. The length of the bladder in the cuff should be equal to 80% of the arm's circumference, and the lower edge of the cuff when positioned should end about one inch above the antecubital fossa (inner elbow). Inflate the cuff to 160 to 180 initially, and increase the pressure if pulse sounds are heard at that level.
- Ask further questions as indicated: This may focus on the primary complaint or others, depending on the situation.
- Conduct a physical examination: Examine the body; palpate for areas of tenderness or swelling; auscultate heart, lung, and abdominal sounds; and note any injuries. Do a brief head-to-toe assessment, and compare one side of the body with the other, noting any asymmetry.
- Treat any life-threatening injuries or conditions noted immediately.

Assessing the Patient's Level of Consciousness

The AVPU is a quick assessment done to determine the patient's level of consciousness. This may be one of the first assessments done when initially attending to a patient.

Alert, voice, pain, unresponsive (AVPU)			
A	Alert and awake; aware of person, place, time, and condition. Follows commands. Pediatric: Active and responds to external stimuli and to caregiver.	Yes	No
V	Responds to verbal stimuli, but the eyes do not open spontaneously. Pediatric: Responds only when the caregiver calls the child's name.	Yes	No
P	Responds to painful stimuli, such as pinching the skin/earlobe, but not to verbal stimuli. Pediatric: Responds only to painful stimuli, such as pinching the nailbed.	Yes	No
U	Unresponsive; does not respond to painful or verbal stimuli. Pediatric: Unresponsive.	Yes	No

Reassessment

Reassessment involves ongoing monitoring of the patient at regular intervals to determine changes in his or her condition or trends such as decreasing BP or increasing agitation. Reassessment is done after a secondary assessment. Unstable patients should be reassessed at least every 5 minutes and stable patients every 15 minutes. Reassessment should include reviewing the primary assessment, taking vital signs, repeating the physical examination (including evaluation of mental status), and monitoring the chief complaint and response to interventions. Reassessment findings should be compared to baseline findings. The patient's airway, ventilation, and circulation should be reassessed as well as the patient's degree of pain—stable, better, or worse. Each intervention should be reassessed for effectiveness and the need for modifications of treatment or if new interventions should be determined. If the patient is receiving oxygen, the tank and all of the equipment should be checked to ensure that they are functioning properly.

Medicine

Circulatory System

The **circulatory system** controls blood flow throughout the body and to the tissues, controls gas exchange (carbon dioxide and oxygen), serves as a reservoir for blood, maintains blood pH through a buffer system, responds to infections, and facilitates coagulation (blood clotting). The circulatory system includes the cardiovascular system (heart and blood vessels) and the blood.

- Heart: Has four chambers, upper (right atrium and left atrium) and lower (right ventricle and left ventricle). The heart muscle receives blood from two major coronary arteries and their branches.
- Vessels: The venous system includes veins, venules, and venous capillaries and brings blood back to the heart via the inferior and superior vena cava. The arterial system, including the coronary arteries, branches from the aorta after it leaves the heart and includes arteries, arterioles, and arterial capillaries.
- Blood: Red blood cells (erythrocytes); white blood cells (leukocytes including monocytes, lymphocytes, basophils, neutrophils, and eosinophils); platelets (thrombocytes); and plasma, the liquid portion of the blood (which contains clotting factors).

The circulatory system is responsible for the oxygenation of cells, perfusion (carrying blood with oxygen, glucose, and nutrients to cells), and removing waste products such as carbon dioxide.

Altered Mental Status

Altered mental status occurs because brain functioning is disrupted. Signs of altered mental status may be subtle (such as slight agitation, lethargy, sleepiness, or forgetfulness) or more obvious (such as disorientation, confusion, personality changes, violent behavior, somnolence, seizures, and coma). An altered mental status may occur abruptly or may have a slower onset, depending on the cause.

- Inadequate oxygenation: Brain cells can only survive about 6 minutes without oxygen, but damage begins to occur after about 60 seconds.
- Inadequate ventilation: Even if oxygen is plentiful, gas exchange is inadequate with impaired ventilation.
- Overdose of medication: May occur with numerous drugs, including opioids/narcotics (such as heroin and oxycodone), antipsychotics, hallucinogens, inhalants, cocaine, methamphetamines, and benzodiazepines.
- Poisoning: Includes arsenic; lead; cyanide; and overdose of medications such as acetaminophen, clonidine, salicylates, calcium channel blockers, and beta blockers.
- Infection: Systemic infections (sepsis), brain abscesses, chronic infections (human immunodeficiency virus/acquired immune deficiency syndrome [HIV/AIDS]).
- Psychological/psychiatric condition: Includes bipolar disorder, schizophrenia, post-traumatic stress disorder (PTSD), and depression.
- Diabetes: Hyperglycemia and hypoglycemia (especially insulin reaction).

Neurological System

The **neurological (nervous) system** consists of the central nervous system ([CNS] brain, spinal cord and nerves) and the peripheral nervous system ([PNS] sensory neurons, ganglia [nerve clusters], and nerves connecting to the CNS). The brain consists of the cerebrum (frontal, temporal, parietal, and occipital lobes); the cerebellum; and the brain stem, which is continuous with the spinal cord. The PNS is divided into the autonomic nervous system (ANS) and the somatic nervous system (SoNS). The autonomic nervous system controls the body's organs and maintains homeostasis (balance). Functions of the ANS include control of the heart rate and function, respiration, digestion, sexual arousal, and other systems. The SoNS comprises cranial and spinal nerves that connect the CNS to the skeletal muscles and skin. The SoNS is the voluntarily controlled component of the PNS, and it receives and responds to external sensory stimuli from the skin and sensory organs.

Ischemic and Hemorrhagic Strokes

Strokes result from interruption of blood flow to an area of the brain. Ischemic strokes (80%) are caused by blockage of an artery supplying the brain, usually from a thrombus (blood clot) or embolus (traveling clot). Hemorrhagic strokes (20%) result from a ruptured cerebral artery, causing not only a lack of oxygen and nutrients but also edema (swelling) that causes widespread pressure and damage. With both types, patients may experience weakness, paralysis, and loss of sensation in one or more extremities; difficulty speaking or loss of speech; vision impairment; difficulty swallowing; headache; an altered state of consciousness (confusion, disorientation); or coma. Transient ischemic attacks (TIAs) from small clots cause similar but short-lived (minutes to hours) symptoms. Emergent treatment includes placing the patient in the semi-Fowlers or Fowler's position and administering oxygen. The patient may require oral suctioning if the secretions pool. The patient's airway, breathing, and circulation should be assessed. Patients should be transported immediately to the receiving facility because thrombolytic therapy to dissolve blood clots should be administered within 1 to 3 hours.

Cincinnati Prehospital Stroke Scale

The Cincinnati Prehospital Stroke Scale should be administered to any patient who is suspected of having a stroke. The patient may be experiencing a stroke if testing positive for any of the three signs and should be transported to the receiving facility as soon as possible.

Cincinnati Prehospital Stroke Scale		
Signs	**Directions to patient**	**Abnormal results**
Facial drooping	Smile. Show your teeth.	One side of the face is weak or paralyzed and doesn't move as well as the other.
Arm drifting	Close your eyes and hold your arms out straight and hold them there for 10 seconds.	One arm doesn't move at all or drifts downward.
Speaking abnormality	Repeat after me: "Don't count your chickens before they are hatched."	Patient slurs words, uses inappropriate words, or is unable to respond.

Los Angeles Prehospital Stroke Screen

The **Los Angeles Prehospital Stroke Screen** is used to assess patients in a prehospital setting who have symptoms that suggest a stroke (such as altered state of consciousness, difficulty speaking, one-sided weakness, or paralysis). The results are positive for stroke if all criteria are met or are unable to be measured and the physical exam shows an unequal response. Note: A patient may still be having a stroke even if all the criteria are not met.

General criteria	Yes	No	Unknown
Age >45	X		
No history of epilepsy or seizures	X		
Onset of symptoms <24 hours	X		
Patient was able to walk before the onset of symptoms	X		
Blood glucose between 60 and 400 mg/dL	X		

Physical criteria	Equal	Right	Left
Facial smile	Normal	Droop	Droop
Grip strength	Normal	Weak or no grip	Weak or no grip
Arm strength	Normal	Drifts or falls down	Drifts or falls down

Types of Headaches

Type of headache	Characteristics	Prehospital
Tension	Steady, constant pressure-like pain usually starting in the forehead, temples, or the back of the neck.	May vary depending on the cause and severity. Manage the patient's airway/ventilation/oxygen supplementation as needed, dim the lights, and place the patient in a position of comfort (usually semi-Fowler's or Fowler's), and apply a cold compress.
Cluster	Unilateral, occurring one to eight times daily, often for several weeks and associated with severe pain in the eye and orbit and radiating to the face and temporal area.	
Migraine	Severe recurring headaches often characterized by a prodrome phase, aura phase, headache phase, and recovery phase.	
Head/Neck trauma related	Vary but may start at neck or shoulders and radiate to the top of the head.	
Bleeding/ Stroke related	Epidural: Sudden severe, intense. Subdural: Progressive headache worsening over time. Subarachnoid: "Thunderclap" severe headache with abrupt onset; it may be worse at the back of the head. Stroke: Tension-type headache with the site of pain relating to the area of injury. Often associated with alterations in mental status and other symptoms, such as weakness, paralysis, nausea and vomiting, and photophobia.	

Seizures

Seizures are sudden, involuntary, abnormal electrical disturbances in the brain that can manifest as alterations of consciousness, spastic tonic and clonic movements, convulsions, and loss of consciousness.

- Tonic-clonic (grand mal): Occurs without warning.
  - Tonic period (10–30 seconds): The eyes roll upward with loss of consciousness, the arms flex, and the body stiffens in symmetric contractions with cyanosis and salivating.
  - Clonic period (usually 30 seconds or longer): Violent rhythmic jerking with contraction and relaxation and sometimes incontinence of urine and feces.

During the seizure, the patient's head and body should be protected from injury but no attempt should be made to insert anything into the mouth or restrain the patient. If possible, the patient should be screened from spectators and turned onto his or her side (the recovery position) to prevent aspiration. Following seizures, there may be confusion, disorientation, and impairment of motor activity and speech and vision for several hours. Headache, nausea, and vomiting may occur. Prehospital: Monitor the airway, breathing, and circulation and suction and administer oxygen as needed. Insert a nasopharyngeal airway for assisted ventilation if the patient is cyanotic.

Partial Seizures

Partial seizures are caused by an electrical discharge to a localized area of the cerebral cortex, such as the frontal, temporal, or parietal lobes with seizure characteristics related to the area of involvement. They may begin in a focal area and become generalized, often preceded by an aura.

- Simple partial: Unilateral motor symptoms including somatosensory, psychic, and autonomic.
  - Aversive: Eyes and head are turned away from the focal side.
  - Sylvan (usually during sleep): Tonic-clonic movements of the face, salivation, and arrested speech.
- Special sensory: Various sensations (numbness, tingling, prickling, or pain) spreading from one area. May include visual sensations, posturing, or hypertonia. These are rare in patients <8 years old.
- Complex (psychomotor): There is no loss of consciousness, but there may be altered levels of consciousness, and patients may be nonresponsive with amnesia. May involve complex sensorium with bad tastes, auditory or visual hallucinations, and a feeling of déjà vu or strong fear. Patients may carry out repetitive activities, such as walking, running, smacking lips, chewing, or drawling. Patients are rarely aggressive. The seizure is usually followed by prolonged drowsiness and confusion. Occurs from age 3 through adolescence.

Prehospital: Provide supportive care.

Status Epilepticus

Status epilepticus (SE) is usually generalized tonic-clonic seizures that are characterized by a series of seizures with the intervening time being too short for the regaining of consciousness. The constant seizures and periods of apnea can lead to exhaustion, respiratory failure with hypoxemia and hypercapnia, hyperthermia, cardiac failure, and death. SE may result from uncontrolled epilepsy, noncompliance with anticonvulsive treatment, stroke, encephalopathy, drug toxicity, brain trauma, brain tumors (neoplasms), and metabolic disorders. SE is life threatening, so treatment should begin as soon as possible.

Prehospital care includes the following:

- Place an intravenous (IV) line.
- If opioid drug intoxication is the suspected cause, administer naloxone.
- Administer midazolam (intramuscular [IM]) (5 to 10 mg), lorazepam (IV), or diazepam (IV) to control seizures.
- Intubate and ventilate if in respiratory distress.
- Provide supportive care for seizures to prevent injury.
- Control hyperthermia with room-temperature water to skin and an IV normal saline (NS) bolus of 500 mL.

Glasgow Coma Scale (GCS)

The **Glasgow Coma Scale (GCS)** measures the depth and duration of coma or impaired levels of consciousness; it is used for postoperative assessment. The GCS measures three parameters: best eye response, best verbal response, and best motor response, with a total possible score that ranges from 3 to 15. The same scale is used with slight modifications for infants.

Eye opening	4: Spontaneous. 3: To verbal stimuli. 2: To pain (not of face). 1: No response.
Verbal	5: Oriented (Infant: Smiles, exhibits appropriate interactions). 4: Conversation is confused, but he or she can answer questions (Infant: Crying but consolable). 3: Uses inappropriate words (Infant: Moaning, sometimes inconsolable). 2: Speech incomprehensible (Infant: Inconsolable, agitated). 1: No response.
Motor	6: Moves on command (Infant: Moves spontaneously or with purpose). 5: Moves purposefully to respond to pain. 4: Withdraws in response to pain. 3: Decorticate posturing (flexion) in response to pain. 2: Decerebrate posturing (extension) in response to pain. 1: No response.

Injuries/conditions are classified according to the total score as follows: 3–8, coma; ≤ 8, severe head injury; 9–12, moderate head injury; 13–15, mild head injury.

Acute Abdomen

Acute abdomen is an acute intra-abdominal disorder that occurs with abrupt onset and usually requires emergency surgical intervention, although some patients may respond to other treatments, such as antibiotics. Acute abdomen may result from infection (peritonitis, pancreatitis, cholecystitis, appendicitis, diverticulitis), perforation, rupture of an internal organ (such as the spleen), aortic aneurysm, obstruction, infarction (necrotic tissue resulting from a blood clot or obstructed blood supply). If the blood supply is interrupted, gangrene may occur within 6 hours. Acute abdomen is characterized by inflammation, distension (often including guarding and rigidity), and acute pain (moderate/severe of fewer than 7 days' duration). Abdominal pain is especially concerning in pediatric and geriatric patients and those with impaired immune systems (such as HIV/AIDS patients and those receiving chemotherapy). Acute abdomen in infants and children may indicate conditions not commonly found in adults such as pyloric stenosis, volvulus, and necrotizing enterocolitis. Prehospital: Obtain a medical history regarding the quality, location, and duration of pain as well as referred pain; place the patient in a comfortable position; administer oxygen; and provide rapid transport.

Gastrointestinal (GI) Tract

Body part	Function
Mouth	Chews, moistens, begins carbohydrate hydrolysis (the breakdown of food by enzymes), creates a bolus of food. Connected to the esophagus by the pharynx.
Esophagus	Transports a bolus through the lower esophageal sphincter (which prevents backflow up the esophagus) to the stomach by peristalsis (wavelike contractions).
Stomach	Churns, secretes acids and enzymes, begins hydrolysis of proteins, and creates chyme (a more fluid substance).
Small intestine (about 20 feet long)	<u>Duodenum:</u> Accepts chyme and digests food to prepare for absorption. <u>Jejunum:</u> Absorbs most of the nutrients from the food, including vitamin B_{12}. Accepts bile from the liver and gallbladder to digest fats and pancreatic enzymes from the pancreas to digest proteins, fats, and carbohydrates. <u>Ileum:</u> Contains the ileocecal valve, which controls the flow of chyme into the large intestine.
Large intestine (about 5 feet long)	<u>Cecum:</u> Reabsorbs fluids and electrolytes. <u>Appendix:</u> Serves no function. <u>Ascending, transverse, descending colon:</u> Reabsorbs water, vitamin K, and electrolytes to form feces.
Rectum	Stores feces.
Anus	Contains sphincters that control the expelling of feces.

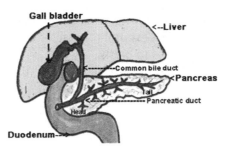

Peritonitis

Peritonitis is a bacterial infection of the peritoneum (lining of the abdominal cavity) that can lead to septicemia and death. Patients with kidney failure (especially those patients on peritoneal dialysis), liver disease, or infection of the GI tract are especially at risk. Other causes include an abdominal wound, ruptured appendix, perforated colon, diverticulitis, abdominal surgery, and inflammatory bowel disease. Symptoms include signs of acute abdomen: abdominal pain and distension, rigid abdomen, nausea and vomiting, diarrhea, fever, and chills. Other symptoms may include decreased urine output, excessive thirst, and tachycardia (rapid pulse). Peritonitis may be associated with ulcerative diseases, such as Crohn's disease (open sores through all layers of the walls of any part of the GI tract, most commonly in the ileum) and ulcerative colitis (open sores in the inner lining of the colon). Prehospital: Obtain an accurate medical history, note the condition of the abdomen with gentle palpation, provide supplemental oxygen/ventilation as needed, and position the patient for comfort because he or she may be experiencing severe pain.

Pediatric and Geriatric Patients with Abdominal Pain

Because **pediatric patients** (infants and small children) have large organs in relation to their size and very little protection with muscles or bone, organs such as the bladder, liver, and kidneys are more likely to suffer injury from abdominal trauma than they are in adults. Children have smaller rib cages and pelvic bones, so the abdomen is more vulnerable. Abdominal pain in children may be associated with constipation (right lower quadrant pain) as well as appendicitis, which is characterized by right lower quadrant pain and a lack of appetite, but it may be hard to identify in children because they may not have appreciable or localized pain initially. Pain persisting for ≥48 hours usually indicates rupture of the appendix. Vomiting and diarrhea may rapidly deplete fluids because of lower fluid volume, resulting in dehydration. **Geriatric patients** with acute abdomen may not exhibit typical abdominal rigidity or guarding. Additionally, abdominal pain may be an indication of a heart attack rather than a GI problem.

Ulcerative Colitis and Crohn's Disease

Ulcerative colitis is superficial inflammation of the mucosa of the colon and rectum, causing ulcerations ranging from pinpoint to extensive. Ulcerations may bleed and produce purulent material. The mucosa of the bowel becomes swollen, erythematous (red), and granular. Onset is usually between ages 15 and 30. Ulcerative colitis may affect only the rectum, the entire colon, or only the left colon. Indications include abdominal pain (usually absent or mild unless disease is severe), bloody diarrhea, rectal bleeding, fecal urgency, and tenesmus (a constant feeling of having to defecate). **Crohn's disease** is chronic inflammation of any area of the GI system but most commonly the small intestine and the beginning of the large intestine, resulting in ulcers that may involve the full thickness of the intestinal wall. An acute flare-up may mimic appendicitis. Indications include diarrhea (watery), rectal bleeding, abdominal cramping and pain (usually in the right lower quadrant), nausea, vomiting, fever, and night sweats. Prehospital: Provide supportive care, manage the patient's airway/ventilation/oxygen supplementation (to maintain oxygen saturation of ≥94%), and provide shock treatment per protocol if necessary.

Allergic Reactions and Anaphylaxis

Allergic reactions are a response of the body's immune system to an antigen (substance), such as peanuts or shellfish. The body produces antibodies (immunoglobulins, such as IgE or non-IgE) that can identify and try to neutralize or destroy antigens. Allergic responses may be mild (local rash, redness, itching, swelling, congestion), moderate (generalized itching, difficulty breathing), or severe (life-threatening anaphylaxis). With **anaphylaxis**, an antigen triggers the release of substances that affect the skin, cardiopulmonary system, and GI system. Histamine causes initial redness and swelling by inducing vasodilation. In some cases, initial reactions may be mild, but subsequent contact can cause severe life-threatening response. Symptoms include the following: a sudden onset of weakness, dizziness, and confusion; tachycardia; generalized swelling; itching; severe low BP leading to shock; airway obstruction; nausea and vomiting; hives; diarrhea; seizures; coma; and death. Prehospital: For hypotension and facial swelling, respiratory distress, or swelling of the mouth, provide epinephrine (if authorized) or assist with an autoinjector to the lateral thigh and repeat every 5–10 minutes as needed, provide supplemental oxygen/ventilation, and transport immediately.

- 63 -

Infectious and Contagious Diseases

Infectious diseases, which may be communicable or noncommunicable, are those that are caused when microorganisms (such as bacteria, viruses, retroviruses, protozoa, helminths [worms] and fungi) invade the body and cause disease. Noncommunicable diseases may spread from an environmental source, such as contaminated water or food (such as with food poisoning), or from insects that carry the disease (such as with Lyme disease). However, they do not spread from person to person, so only standard precautions are needed when caring for these patients. Contagious diseases are infections that are communicable from person to person. They may be spread through direct physical contact and sneezing or coughing as well as through contact with blood or other body fluids (feces, semen, urine, or perspiration). With contagious diseases, the type of precautions needed depends on the mode of infection and they may range from contact to droplet to airborne precautions; the type of PPE needed also varies.

Decontaminating an Ambulance

Decontaminating an ambulance begins with removal of any debris, with sharps being deposited in a sharps container and soiled linen being red-bagged. Then, the equipment and surfaces that have had contact with a patient or with contaminated materials must be cleaned, disinfected, or sterilized, depending on the type of equipment/surface and the type of contamination. Between patients, surfaces and equipment should be wiped down with a disinfectant, such as a 1:100 bleach solution or premixed wipes. Alcohol-based products are effective for many organisms, but not for *Clostridium difficile* (which is spread through fecal contamination). If equipment is left with a patient at a receiving facility, that facility must clean the equipment or place it in a red bag before returning it. At the end of the day, the entire ambulance should be cleaned. Various methods of sterilization, including the use of a fogging agent and UV lights, are available. All cleaning procedures must be recorded for compliance purposes.

Gastrointestinal (GI) Bleeding

Upper **GI bleeding** (mouth to stomach) is characterized by nausea and hematemesis (vomiting of bright-red blood or partially digested, dark-brown, granulated ["coffee ground"] blood) and/or abdominal pain on palpation. With lower GI bleeding (small intestine to anus), the abdomen may be distended and tender and the patient may be passing blood through the anus. If bleeding has been slow and chronic, the patient may have only vague complaints of weakness and abdominal discomfort. In all cases, blood will mix with the stool. Melena (black-colored stool) usually indicates an upper GI bleed because the blood has been partially digested. Hematochezia (wine-colored stool or bright-red blood in the stool) indicates a lower GI bleed. Patients develop shock if blood loss is profound ($\geq 40\%$). Prehospital: Examine the abdomen and note pain, monitor vital signs, and note signs of acute blood loss (fall in BP; increase in pulse; pallor; or cold, clammy skin). Provide suctioning if needed. Provide supplemental oxygen and ventilation as needed. Place the patient in the recovery position if he or she is vomiting. Place the patient flat with the feet elevated for shock.

Endocrine Disorders

Diabetic Conditions

Diabetes mellitus is a group of metabolic disorders that involve hyperglycemia (increased blood glucose [sugar]) because of defective production and/or action of insulin. Insulin metabolizes glucose to produce energy as fuel for body cells.

- Type 1: Autoimmune destruction of beta cells in the pancreas results in no or deficient insulin production. Treatment: Insulin. Symptoms: Rapid onset, increased thirst, frequent urination, increased hunger, delayed healing, weight loss, frequent infections, and blurred vision.
- Type 2: Insulin baseline may be normal or deficient, but there is no or an inadequate increase in response to a meal, so the glucose level rises but there is decreased uptake by the tissues. Insulin resistance occurs because there is decreased sensitivity to insulin by the tissues. Type 2 diabetes is often related to obesity. Treatment is with oral diabetic agents. Symptoms include slow onset, increased thirst, increased urination, candidal (fungal) infections, delayed healing, and weight gain.
- Gestational: Beta cells in the pancreas are unable to produce adequate insulin during pregnancy, but normal production resumes after delivery. Treatment varies. Symptoms include being asymptomatic or having increased thirst and urinary frequency.

Pediatric patients with diabetes mellitus most commonly have type 1 and are insulin dependent with the peak age for onset happening during adolescence; however, rates of type 2 diabetes are increasing in young children and adolescents, especially if they are overweight. Children (especially <15) with late stages of hyperglycemia may develop cerebral edema with headache and weakness and changes in mental status, particularly irritability. Children are also more likely to develop hypoglycemia than are adults and are more prone to having seizures and becoming dehydrated than are adults. Hypoglycemia may result from excessive exercise. Many children may be undiagnosed and may present with diabetic ketoacidosis. **Geriatric patients** often have reduced sensation because of neuropathy associated with diabetes, and they may be unaware of injuries. Geriatric patients are also prone to developing dehydration and infections. Diabetes is the leading cause of lower limb amputation and kidney failure, so many patients with amputations and on hemodialysis are diabetic. Patients with diabetes may have an atypical presentation of a myocardial infarction (heart attack) without chest pain.

Hyperglycemia

Hyperglycemia is high blood glucose (sugar) with a level of greater than 130mg/dL after fasting for 8 hours or greater than 180 mg/dL 2 hours after eating. Hyperglycemia may occur in undiagnosed diabetic patients or in diabetic patients who have taken inadequate insulin; those who have eaten a diet too high in carbohydrates (sugars); or those who are ill, such as with an infection. Initial signs include polyuria (increased urine), polyphagia (hunger), polydipsia (increased thirst), headaches, lethargy, fatigue, and blurred vision, but if blood sugar is very high (greater than 250 mg/dL), then patients may become increasingly somnolent, and the patient may develop diabetic ketoacidosis from the buildup of ketones as fat is broken down by the body for energy because sugar/glucose cannot be used. The patient may exhibit Kussmaul's breathing (fruity-smelling breath from ketones), could lapse into a coma, and could die if left untreated. Prehospital: Question the patient about diabetes and the use of diabetic medications. Check the patient's blood sugar level; monitor the vital signs and oxygen saturation, and provide supportive care as needed. Rapid transport is required with altered levels of consciousness.

Hyperglycemic Hyperosmolar Nonketotic Syndrome (HHNS) or Coma (HHNK)

Hyperglycemic hyperosmolar nonketotic syndrome (HHNS) or **coma (HHNK)** occurs in people without a history of diabetes or in people with mild type 2 diabetes but with insulin resistance resulting in persistent hyperglycemia, which causes osmotic diuresis. Fluid shifts from intracellular to extracellular spaces to maintain osmotic equilibrium, but the increased glycosuria and dehydration result in hypernatremia and increased osmolality (concentration). This condition is most common in persons 50–70 years old, and it often is precipitated by an acute illness such as a stroke, medications such as thiazides, or dialysis treatments. HHNS differs from ketoacidosis because although the insulin level is not adequate, it is high enough to prevent the breakdown of fat. Symptoms include polyuria, dehydration, hypotension, tachycardia, blood glucose >500 mg/dL, changes in mental status, hallucinations, seizures, and hemiparesis. Prehospital: Question the patient about his or her history of diabetes and use of diabetes medications. Check the patient's blood sugar level, monitor the vital signs and oxygen saturation, and provide supportive care as needed. Rapid transport is needed for altered levels of consciousness.

Hypoglycemia

Hypoglycemia (low blood sugar/glucose) is most often caused by an insulin reaction (too much insulin for the amount of glucose/sugar intake) or an overdose of oral diabetes medications, which stimulate the overproduction of insulin. Hypoglycemia may occur if patients took insulin but skipped a meal, vomited, or exercised too strenuously, depleting the body of sugar/glucose while insulin levels remain high. Increased insulin levels cause glucose levels to fall to at or below 70 mg/dL, initially resulting in tremors, headache, blurred vision dizziness, and pallor leading to confusion, bizarre behavior, lack of coordination, combative behavior, personality changes, tachycardia, and irregular heartbeat. Severe hypoglycemia may lead to seizures, coma, and death. Hypoglycemia is life threatening if untreated. Infants may have dehydration and seizures; geriatric patients may have dehydration and stroke. Prehospital: Ask the patient about his or her diabetes status and use of diabetes medications. Check the patient's glucose level, and administer oral glucose tablets, one tablespoon of sugar, or a glass of orange juice if the patient is able to swallow; provide rapid transport for altered levels of consciousness.

Assessment of Psychiatric Patients

Assessment of patients with psychological/psychiatric symptoms should begin with a history that includes the patient's age and cultural/spiritual background and whether the patient has experienced similar symptoms previously or has a history of a psychiatric disorder as well as any history of substance abuse. Assessment includes the following:

- General appearance: Note hygiene, grooming, appropriate dress, eye contact, unusual movements (twitching, posturing, repetitive movements), and the appearance and condition of the skin.
- Speech: Note speech cadence and abnormal word use, such as neologisms (invented words), clang associations (rhyming), word salad (string of random words), and associative looseness (ideas shifting from one to another).
- Posture/Gait: Note automatisms (purposeless behaviors, such as drumming fingers), slowed motions, waxy flexibility (maintaining an awkward position for extended periods of time), ability to walk, and abnormalities of gait.

- Mental status: Note the patient's state of being alert versus nonalert, responsive versus nonresponsive, and coherent versus noncoherent; clarity of ideas; suicidal ideation; and desire for self-harm.
- Mood and affect: Note facial expressions, expressed emotions, and affect (blunted, broad, flat, inappropriate, restricted).
- Memory/Intellectual processes: Note if memory and intellectual processes are intact or impaired. Is the patient disoriented and confused or alert and responsive?
- Attention: Note if the patient's attention is focused or unfocused.

Behavioral Alterations

Behavioral alterations may include agitation, anger, throwing temper tantrums (children), acting aggressively (adolescents/adult), exhibiting poor judgment, and acting inappropriately. Behavioral alterations may result from psychiatric disorders (such as depression, schizophrenia, and bipolar disorder) and psychiatric medications as well as numerous other causes, including the following:

- Hypoglycemia/Low blood sugar (insulin reaction).
- Lack of adequate oxygen interferes with brain function.
- Shock (low BP; a rapid pulse results in inadequate blood supply to the brain).
- Mind-altering substances (cocaine, methamphetamine, lysergic acid diethylamide [LSD], Rohypnol [the date-rape drug]).
- Brain infection (meningitis, encephalitis, brain abscess).
- Seizure disorders (epilepsy, other causes of seizures).
- Poisoning/Overdose (lead poisoning, drug overdose).
- Malnutrition resulting in inadequate nourishment of brain tissue.
- Substance abuse (drug or alcohol abuse/withdrawal).
- Heat extremes (hypothermia/hyperthermia).

Indications of being a danger to self or others include severe agitation, hallucinations, delusional thinking, paranoia, self-destructive behavior (cutting, drug/alcohol abuse, promiscuity, risk-taking activities), depression, and suicide attempts. A patient may pose a risk to others if he or she is behaving in a threatening or violent manner and has a weapon (club, gun, knife, baseball bat).

Calming Patients with Behavioral Emergencies

Patients with **behavioral emergencies** are often agitated and may be confused, fearful, and/or aggressive, so the EMT must remain calm and approach the patient slowly; remain at a safe distance; and avoid fast movements, threatening postures, or attempts at physical contact, acknowledging the patient's agitation and offering assistance ("I can see that you're upset, and I want to help") and maintaining eye contact (unless the person is violent and reacts aggressively). The EMT should encourage the patient to talk about what is causing the behavior and should answer questions honestly while avoiding threatening, arguing, or challenging the patient. If the patient is suffering hallucinations or delusional thinking, the EMT should avoid playing along ("I don't see what you do") but should also avoid contradicting the patient directly when responding. Family or friends may assist with intervention. The EMT should not leave the patient unattended and should try to lower distressing stimuli (such as lights and noise) and consider contacting law enforcement. Restraints should be avoided if possible.

Suicidal Ideation

Suicidal ideation occurs frequently in those with mood disorders or depression (common in geriatric patients). Although females are more likely to attempt suicide, males actually successfully commit suicide three times more often than females, primarily because females tend to take overdoses from which they can be revived whereas males choose more violent means (jumping from a high place, shooting, or hanging). This holds true for adolescents and adults. Risk factors include psychiatric disorders (schizophrenia, bipolar disorder, post-traumatic stress disorder [PTSD], and substance abuse), physical disorders (HIV/AIDS, diabetes, traumatic brain injury, spinal cord injury), and social problems (bullying). Passive suicidal ideation involves wishing to be dead or thinking about dying without making plans, whereas active suicidal ideation involves making plans. Patients at risk should be questioned about their feelings, problems, plans for suicide, and access to weapons. High-risk findings include the following:

- Violent suicide attempt (knives, gunshots) or access to a weapon.
- History of a suicide attempt and a suicide attempt with a low chance of rescue.
- Ongoing psychosis or disordered thinking.
- Ongoing severe depression and feelings of helplessness.
- Lack of a social support system.

Agitated/Excited Delirium

Patients with **agitated/excited delirium** are often very combative, aggressive, violent, and uncooperative, and they exhibit shouting, threaten violence, and behave bizarrely. The patient may experience hallucinations, disorientation, paranoia, and panic. Patients may be exceptionally strong and seem insensitive to pain. They are often hyperthermic (high temperature). Agitated/Excited delirium may be associated with hypoglycemia, brain damage, chemical imbalance, and substance abuse (methamphetamine, cocaine, phencyclidine [PCP, "angel dust"], and LSD). Patients often require restraints for their own or for others' safety, but they are at risk of death by asphyxiation or restraint (positional) because they fight desperately against the restraints. Prehospital: The EMT should use active listening and try to establish rapport while assessing the patient's intellectual functioning, orientation, judgment and thought processes, language, mood, and appearance to determine if law enforcement or other assistance is needed. The patient may refuse care, but implied consent is legal for patients with abnormal behavior. The patient must be transported safely for treatment. The EMT should look for medications or drugs on site and take them to the receiving facility.

Restraints

Patients needing restraints are often agitated, confused, and refuse care, but implied consent is legal for patients with abnormal behavior. **Restraints** include the following:

- <u>Verbal:</u> Try to calm the patient while being firm.
- <u>Nonverbal:</u> Use body language and a show of force (with a number of EMS personnel being present) to convince the patient.
- <u>Physical:</u> Use standard precautions; one person is assigned to each limb, while a fifth person reassures and tries to calm the patient. Apply multiple restraints as necessary, including across the trunk, being careful not to restrict the patient's breathing.
- <u>Chemical:</u> Use as a last resort (usually after physical restraints). Includes benzodiazepines (lorazepam) and neuroleptics (haloperidol).

- Tasers/Electrical stun guns: These may be used by law enforcement to subdue a severely agitated patient. They may cause burns, dart injuries, fall injuries, or cardiac arrest. Stun guns require direct contact, but Tasers may be shot from 20 feet away.

Document the reason for restraint, the types of restraints, the restraint technique, and the time the patient is restrained. Monitor the patient's condition continuously, including the heart rate, airway/ventilation/oxygen supplementation, and circulation.

Circulatory System

The **circulatory system** is responsible for the oxygenation of cells, perfusion (carrying of blood with oxygen, glucose, and nutrients to the cells), and gas exchange (removing waste products, such as carbon dioxide). The circulatory system serves as a blood reservoir (5 L), maintains blood pH (7.35–7.45) through a buffer system, responds to infections, and facilitates coagulation (blood clotting). The heart is located between the lungs and under and to the left of the mediastinum (breastbone). The heart has four chambers: upper (right atrium, left atrium) and lower (right ventricle and left ventricle). The myocardium (heart muscle) receives blood from two major coronary arteries and their branches. The inner lining of the heart is the endocardium, and the lining that surrounds the heart is the pericardium, which has an inner double-layered serous membrane (visceral pericardium) and a fibrous outer layer (parietal pericardium). The cardiac cycle involves one complete heartbeat with systole (ventricular contraction) and diastole (relaxation) phases. Stroke volume is the volume of blood ejected from the left ventricle in one cardiac cycle (about 60–70 mL), and cardiac output is the heart rate times the stroke volume.

The venous system includes the veins, venules, and venous capillaries, and it brings blood back to the heart via the inferior and superior vena cava. The arterial system includes the coronary arteries, which branch from the aorta after it leaves the heart; arteries; arterioles; and arterial capillaries. **The blood flows** as follows:

- Deoxygenated venous blood returns to the heart per the inferior vena cava, superior vena cava, and coronary sinus (bringing blood from the coronary arteries) into the right atrium, and then it flows through the tricuspid valve into the right ventricle.
- From the right ventricle, blood flows through the pulmonic (semilunar) valve into the pulmonary artery and to the lungs to exchange carbon dioxide for oxygen.
- Oxygenated blood flows from the lungs through the pulmonary veins into the left atrium and through the mitral (bicuspid) valve into the left ventricle.
- From the left ventricle, blood flows through the aortic valve and into the aorta, the coronary arteries, and the general circulation through the thoracic and abdominal aorta.

After blood flows through the valves, they close to prevent backflow. Both atria and both ventricles contract simultaneously.

Components of the Blood

Blood cells are produced in the bone marrow. Blood is a viscous, dark-red fluid comprised of cells, gases, and plasma (55%). Blood components include the following:

- Erythrocytes (red blood cells [RBCs]): RBCs carry hemoglobin, which transports oxygen. If the RBC count is low (such as from blood loss) or the oxygen-carrying capacity is impaired (such as with anemia), the patient may experience hypoxemia (low oxygen). The life cycle of RBCs is normally 120 days.

- Leukocytes (white blood cells [WBCs]): WBCs defend the body against invading organisms (viruses, bacteria, fungi, and parasites), and in the bloodstream and tissues they respond to allergies. WBCs include lymphocytes (B, T, natural killer, and null cells), monocytes, eosinophils, basophils, and neutrophils.
- Thrombocytes (platelets): Platelets release clotting factors and have an active role in forming blood clots.
- Plasma (55% of blood): Plasma carries water, proteins, electrolytes, lipids (fats), blood cells, and glucose as well as clotting factors.

The primary blood types are A, B, AB, and O. Blood is either Rh– or RH+, and patients must receive transfusions of blood that are type and Rh compatible.

Angina and Heart Attack

Chest pain may indicate angina (pain from temporary constriction/blockage of blood flow in the coronary arteries) or a heart attack (pain caused by blockage of blood flow to the heart muscle because of a blood clot [most common] or hemorrhage, resulting in the death of heart tissue). Heart problems in children are often associated with congenital heart disease. Geriatric and female patients may not have chest pain with a heart attack. Make note of the following:

- Character, location, and severity of the pain.
- Radiation of pain to the neck, jaw, arms, back, jaw, and/or stomach.
- Shortness of breath at rest or with exertion or worsening when lying flat.
- Skin: Cold, clammy skin is common with a heart attack.
- Vital signs: Note BP, pulse (rapid, irregular, slow), and respirations.
- Other: Note nausea and/or vomiting and dizziness/lightheadedness.

Prehospital: Provide the patient with a position of comfort (often semi-Fowler's if there is shortness of breath), provide a high concentration of oxygen with a nonrebreather mask, question the patient about medications taken recently and/or medications taken for pain (such as aspirin or nitroglycerin), and provide rapid transport.

Perfusion, Oxygenation of Tissues, and Cardiac Compromise

Perfusion depends on an adequate supply of red blood cells, which carry oxygen. Perfusion may be impaired if the heart does not pump adequately, if the rate of heart contractions is too low or too rapid to be effective, and if the volume of blood and/or red blood cells pumped is not adequate to provide oxygenation to the tissues. With adequate perfusion, **oxygenation of tissues** occurs when blood flows throughout the body, and gas exchange of carbon dioxide and waste products for oxygen occurs at the capillaries. **Cardiac compromise** results in inadequate circulation and/or perfusion of vital organs. Cardiac compromise may result from atherosclerosis (plaques/fatty deposits) in the arterial lumens, resulting in obstructed blood flow and inadequate dilation and constriction of arteries. Ischemia (low oxygenation) occurs with decreased blood flow and can damage tissues, but occlusion (obstruction) can result in the death of tissue. Cardiac compromise may result from heart damage causing an inadequate heart rate and/or pumping. Cardiac compromise may also result from an inadequate volume of circulating blood.

Management of a Patient with Chest Pain

Management of a patient with chest pain begins with a thorough assessment, primary and secondary survey, and use of the OPQRST and SAMPLE methods of history taking. Patients are often very frightened, so the EMT should provide clear feedback and reassurance. The patient should be placed in the semi-Fowler's position, especially if he or she is experiencing shortness of breath, and the oxygen saturation should be monitored. Respiratory compromise may require supplemental oxygen, bag-mask ventilation (BVM) assistance, PEEP, CPAP/BiPAP, manually triggered ventilators (MTVs), or automatic transport ventilators (ATVs). The EMT should determine the need for the assistance of an advanced emergency medical technician (AEMT) or a paramedic.

Pharmacological interventions (assist the patient with medication administration, or administer the medication according to protocol) may include the following:

- Aspirin (for suspected heart attack; Bayer, Heartline, ZORprin, Empirin): Provide 162 to 325 mg chewable (preferred). Contraindicated with GI bleeding, stroke.
- Nitroglycerin (for suspected angina; Nitro-Dur, Nitrolingual, NitroMist): Provide 0.4 mg sublingually repeated every 3–5 minutes up to three doses. Contraindicated if the patient has recently taken Viagra, had a stroke, or has excessive bleeding.
- Oral glucose (for suspected hypoglycemia/insulin reaction): Glucose tablets, solution.

All patients with chest pain should be transported because even mild chest discomfort may indicate that the patient is having a heart attack, especially in older patients and female patients, who often have atypical symptoms.

Cardiogenic Shock

Cardiogenic shock in adults is usually secondary to myocardial infarction damage of >40% of the left ventricle, reducing contractibility, interfering with the pumping mechanism of the heart, and decreasing oxygen perfusion. Characteristics include increased preload, increased afterload, and decreased contractibility. Together, these result in decreased cardiac output and an increase in systemic vascular resistance (SVR) to compensate and protect the vital organs. As the cardiac output decreases, tissue perfusion decreases, coronary artery perfusion decreases, fluid backs up, and the left ventricle fails to adequately pump the blood, resulting in pulmonary edema and right ventricular failure. Indications: Hypotension with systolic BP <90 mm Hg; tachycardia >100 beat/min with weak, thready pulse and dysrhythmias; decreased heart sounds; chest pain; tachypnea and basilar rales; pallor; and cool, moist skin. Prehospital: Manage the patient's airway/ventilation/oxygenation/intubation as needed; install an IV access line with fluid resuscitation; monitor the electrocardiogram (ECG), vital signs, and cardiac status; and provide inotropic/vasopressor (norepinephrine, dopamine) support.

Hypertensive Crisis

Hypertensive crisis (aka malignant hypertension) is a marked elevation in BP that can cause severe organ damage if left untreated. Causes include encephalopathy, intracranial hemorrhage, aortic dissection, eclampsia, and heart failure. Classifications are as follows:

- **Hypertensive emergency**: Acute hypertension, usually >120 mm Hg diastolic; it must be treated immediately to lower the BP in order to prevent damage to vital organs, such as the heart, brain, or kidneys.
- **Hypertensive urgency**: Acute hypertension must be treated within a few hours, but the vital organs are not in immediate danger. The blood pressure is lowered more slowly to avoid hypotension, ischemia of vital organs, or failure of autoregulation with a one-third reduction in 6 hours.

Symptoms include headache, dizziness, dyspnea, weakness, visual disturbances, anxiety, chest pain (atypical), heart failure, acute coronary syndrome, and stroke. Prehospital: Asymptomatic hypertension requires referral to a physician, whereas severe symptoms require rapid transport. Interventions include airway support/ventilation with oxygen supplementation and advanced life support as needed. Patients with severe dyspnea and pulmonary edema may need CPAP.

Angina Pectoris (Stable)

Impairment of blood flow through the coronary arteries leads to ischemia of the cardiac muscle and **angina pectoris**—pain that may occur in the sternum, chest, neck, arms (especially the left arm), or back. The pain frequently occurs with crushing pain substernally, radiating down the left arm or both arms, although this type of pain is more common in males than females, whose symptoms may appear less acute and may include nausea, shortness of breath, and fatigue. Elderly or diabetic patients may also have pain in their arms, no pain at all (silent ischemia), or weakness and numbness in both arms. Stable angina episodes usually last for <5 minutes and are fairly predictable exercise-induced episodes caused by atherosclerotic lesions blocking >75% of the lumen of the affected coronary artery. Precipitating events include exercise; a decrease in the environmental temperature; heavy eating; strong emotions (such as fright or anger); or exertion, including coitus. Stable angina episodes usually resolve in less than 5 minutes by decreasing the activity level and administering sublingual nitroglycerin. Provide supportive care, oxygen, and assist the patient to take nitroglycerin if available.

Angina Pectoris (Unstable, Variant/Prinzmetal's)

Unstable angina (also known as preinfarction or crescendo angina) is a progression of coronary artery disease, and it occurs when there is a change in the pattern of stable angina. The pain may increase, may not respond to a single nitroglycerin dose, and may persist for >5 minutes. Usually pain is more frequent, lasts longer, and may occur at rest when sitting or lying down. Unstable angina may indicate a rupture of an atherosclerotic plaque and the beginning of thrombus formation, so it should always be treated as a medical emergency with rapid transport because it may indicate a myocardial infarction. **Variant angina** (also known as Prinzmetal's angina) results from spasms of the coronary arteries; can be associated with or without atherosclerotic plaques; and is often related to smoking, alcohol, or illicit stimulants. Variant angina frequently occurs cyclically at the same time each day and often while the person is at rest. Nitroglycerin or calcium channel blockers are used for treatment. Prehospital: Provide supportive care and oxygen, and assist the patient to take nitroglycerin if available.

Myocardial Infarction (MI—Heart Attack)

Myocardial infarction (MI—heart attack) may occur after an episode of unstable angina caused by a rupture of an atherosclerotic plaque and thrombosis associated with coronary artery spasm, but it may also result from vasoconstriction, acute blood loss, decreased oxygen, and ingestion of cocaine. Symptoms may vary considerably, with males having the more "classic" symptom of a sudden onset of crushing chest pain. Elderly and diabetic patients may complain primarily of weakness. Symptoms include the following:

- Angina with pain in the chest that may radiate to the neck or arms, crushing pain, tightness (often more than 30 minutes and unrelieved by rest or nitroglycerin).
- Hypertension or hypotension.
- Palpitations, tachycardia, bradycardia, and dysrhythmias.
- Dyspnea.

- ECG changes (ST segment and T-wave changes), tachycardia, bradycardia, and dysrhythmias.
- Pulmonary edema, peripheral edema, weak/absent peripheral pulses.
- Nausea and vomiting.
- Pallor, cold and clammy skin, diaphoresis.
- Neurological/psychological disturbances: Anxiety, light-headedness, headache, visual abnormalities, slurred speech, and fear.

Prehospital: Manage the patient's airway/ventilation/oxygen supplementation, provide supportive care, perform CPR/defibrillation if needed, and provide rapid transport.

Poisoning

Ingestion	Drugs, overdose, toxic/caustic liquids (bleach, cleaning solution, antifreeze, gasoline), mouse/rat poison, pesticides, some plants, and alcohol	Wide range of symptoms, depending on the substance: anaphylaxis, lethargy, constricted pupils, mouth burns, nausea and vomiting, pain, diarrhea, difficulty breathing, confusion, seizures, and coma. (Toddlers are particularly at risk.)
Inhalation	Toxic gases, smoke, hair spray, carbon monoxide, chlorine, halogens	Difficulty breathing, lethargy, confusion, nausea, vomiting, headache, cyanosis, seizures, slurred speech, and coma.
Injection	Heroin, morphine, drug overdose	Local irritation, lethargy, confusion, slurred speech, nausea, vomiting, difficulty breathing, seizures, and coma. (Adolescents are prone to experimentation with drugs.)
Absorption	Cleaning products, various chemicals	Local irritation, anaphylaxis, burns, tissue damage, rash, nausea, vomiting, shortness of breath, and confusion.

Prehospital: Treatment varies according to the severity. Contact a poison control center if necessary, provide supportive care, remove the substance residue from the patient's mouth, place the patient in the recovery position, manage the patient's airway/ventilation/oxygen supplementation, provide CPR as necessary, induce vomiting or administer activated charcoal only if advised by the poison control center or another expert, and provide rapid transport. If the contamination is by inhalation, remove patient from the source as soon as possible. If the contamination is by absorption, remove the contaminated clothes and wash the patient's skin with large amounts of soap and water and flush the affected eyes with water or NS.

Nerve Agents/Cholinergics

Nerve agents/Cholinergics are toxic chemicals (organophosphates) that damage the nervous system and bodily functions, leading to death in a short time. Nerve agents include tabun (GA), sarin (GB), soman (GD), and VX, and they are used in terrorist attacks. GA, BG, and GD persist in the environment for 10 minutes to 24 hours during the summer and 2 hours to 3 days during the winter (cold weather), and they have very fast action. VX persists longer in the environment and is more lethal. Symptoms of exposure (gas/aerosol) include salivation, lacrimation, urination, defecation, GI upset, and emesis (SLUDGE); runny nose; pupil contraction; vision impairment; slurred speech; chest pain; hallucinations; respiratory distress; and coma. High doses may cause immediate seizures and death. Prehospital: Move away from the area quickly or shelter in place, remove the patient's clothing, and wash the patient's body with large amounts of soap and water. Use an autoinjector for atropine and pralidoxime (separate injections [Mark I] or combined dose [DuoDote]), unless there is only mild tearing or a runny nose, and use diazepam for seizures. Provide airway/ventilation/oxygen supplementation and circulation support.

Carbon Monoxide Poisoning

Carbon monoxide poisoning occurs when people breathe in carbon monoxide, usually related to industrial or household accidents or suicide attempts. Carbon monoxide binds to hemoglobin 200 times more readily than oxygen, and once the carbon monoxide binds to hemoglobin (creating carboxyhemoglobin), the hemoglobin can no longer bind to or transport oxygen, resulting in hypoxemia. Symptoms vary depending on the percentage of saturation with carbon monoxide. At 10%, patients may complain of headache and nausea. At >20%, a patient becomes increasingly weak and confused with alterations in mental status. At >30%, a patient may have dyspnea, chest pain, and increased confusion. When the level continues to increase, a patient may experience seizures, coma, and death. The patient's skin color may be cyanotic, pink, or bright cherry red (but this is not a reliable sign). Prehospital: Administer 100% oxygen with a nonrebreather mask and transport.

Poison Control Resources

The **National Capital Poison Center** provides a website with an online tool—webPOISONCONTROL—(https://triage.webpoisoncontrol.org/#/exclusions) and a telephone number (1-800-222-1222) for people who swallow or come into contact (absorbed, inhaled, injected) with poisonous (toxic) substances.

- webPOISONCONTROL: Can be used for patients (ages 6 months to 79 years and nonpregnant women) who are asymptomatic and unintentionally swallowed a single drug or medication, household product, or berries over a short period of time (minutes to a few hours) and are otherwise healthy.
- Telephone contact: Is used for all other situations, including a patient with symptoms, pregnant women, nonswallowing contact, those ages <6 months or >79, or those who swallowed materials or substances other than those listed for online assistance. Telephone contact can be made for any poisoning if it is preferred to online assistance.

This service is free and usually requires about 3 minutes for a response. When calling, be prepared to describe the substance (include the product name and dosage for medications), amount swallowed, age of patient, weight of patient, time since exposure, and the patient's ZIP Code and email address. If unsure of the amount of poison or the weight of the victim, estimates are acceptable.

Autoinjectors

Autoinjectors are spring-loaded syringe/needle devices that contain preloaded doses of medication and can be easily administered by following the directions on the devices. Autoinjectors are available for nerve agent treatment for emergency medical personnel—Mark I and DuoDote.

- Atropine autoinjector: For symptoms of nerve damage (increases heart rate, dries secretions, dilates pupils, and reduces GI upset).
- Pralidoxime (2-PAM chloride) autoinjector: For symptoms of nerve damage, twitching, and difficulty breathing.
- Diazepam autoinjector: For convulsions associated with nerve agents.

Wear appropriate PPE, remove the safety cap, cleanse the skin with alcohol, and (holding the device perpendicular to the skin) apply firm pressure with the tip of the injector against the skin in the outer thigh until the device fires the needle into the muscle tissue (avoid jabbing). Then, hold the autoinjector in place for at least 10 seconds to ensure that the medication is completely injected. Carefully remove the needle from the skin. Avoid touching the needle, and do not attempt to recap it. Dispose of the intact device in a sharps container.

Age-Related Concerns Related to Toxicology

Age-related concerns related to toxicology include the following:

- Toddlers are at risk of ingestion of toxic substances because their taste buds are not yet fully developed and this allows them to drink foul-tasting substances, such as cleaning supplies, which may be kept under a sink where a child has easy access if the cabinet is not secured. Household substances that pose a substantial risk include perfumes, cosmetics, and alcohol. Toddlers may also ingest unsecured medications.
- Adolescents, who often experiment with drugs and alcohol, are at risk from alcohol poisoning and overdose or severe reaction to illicit drugs. Additionally, adolescents often attempt suicide with acetaminophen (Tylenol), sometimes to gain attention, without realizing that it can cause liver failure and death even after resuscitation.
- Geriatric patients are most at risk from medication errors, such as taking the wrong medication, taking medications belonging to friends or family, or taking the wrong dose of a medication.

Substance Abuse

Many people with **substance abuse** (alcohol or drugs) are reluctant to disclose this information. Common agents include cannabis (marijuana), hallucinogens (LSD), stimulants (cocaine, methamphetamine), barbiturates (secobarbital [Seconal], amobarbital [Amytal]), sedatives (zolpidem [Ambien], eszopiclone [Lunesta]), hypnotics/benzodiazepines (alprazolam [Xanax], diazepam [Valium], lorazepam [Ativan]), and opiates (heroin, morphine, fentanyl, oxycodone, hydrocodone). A number of indicators are suggestive of substance abuse.

Physical signs	Other signs
Needle tracks on arms or legs	Odor of alcohol/marijuana on clothing or
Burns on fingers or lips	breath
Pupils abnormally dilated or constricted, eyes watery	Labile emotions, including mood swings, agitation, and anger
Slurring of speech, slow speech	Inappropriate, impulsive, and/or risky
Lack of coordination, instability of gait	behavior
Tremors	Lying
Sniffing repeatedly, nasal irritation	Missing appointments
Persistent cough	Difficulty concentrating/short-term memory
Weight loss	loss, disoriented/confused
Dysrhythmias (abnormal pulse)	Blackouts
Pallor, puffiness of face	Insomnia or excessive sleeping
	Lack of personal hygiene

Ethanol (Alcohol) Abuse and Withdrawal

Ethanol (alcohol that is found in alcoholic beverages, flavorings, and some medications) is a multisystem toxin and CNS depressant. It is often the drug of choice of teenagers, young adults, and those >60 years old. Ethanol overdose affects the CNS and other organs. If patients are easily aroused, they can usually safely sleep off the effects, but if a patient is semiconscious or unconscious, emergency medical treatment is needed. Young children frequently ingest alcohol in products such as perfumes and cleaning solutions, which are often more toxic than alcoholic beverages.

Infants/Young children	Teenagers/Adults
Seizures, coma, death	Altered mental status, coma, circulatory collapse, death
Respiratory depression and hypoxia	Hypotension, bradycardia with arrhythmias
Hypoglycemia (especially infants and toddlers)	Respiratory depression and hypoxia
Hypothermia	Cold, clammy skin or flushed skin
	Acute pancreatitis/abdominal pain

Chronic abuse of ethanol (alcoholism) is associated with alcohol withdrawal syndrome (delirium tremens) with abrupt cessation of alcohol intake, resulting in hallucinations, tachycardia, diaphoresis, sometimes psychotic behavior, and a high mortality rate. Prehospital: Manage the patient's airway/ventilation/oxygen supplementation and provide CPR if necessary, maintain body temperature, and reduce noise/light.

Nonnarcotic Medication Overdose

Drug	Overdose symptoms
Acetaminophen (Tylenol)	Toxicity occurs with dosage >140 mg/kg in one dose or >7.5g in 24 hours: (Initial) Minor gastrointestinal upset. (Days 2–3) Hepatotoxicity (liver damage) with right upper quadrant pain. (Days 3–4) Hepatic failure with metabolic acidosis, coagulopathy, kidney failure, encephalopathy, nausea, vomiting, and possible death. (Days 5–12) Recovery period (survivors). Prehospital: Manage the patient's airway/ventilation/oxygen supplementation. Use the recovery position if the patient is nauseated. Provide supportive care.
NSAIDs/Salicylates	Toxicity (4 to 48 hours after ingestion) includes headache, nausea, abdominal pain, tinnitus (ringing in the ears), diaphoresis, hypertension, fluid in the lungs, alterations in mental status, cardiac dysrhythmias, seizures, and respiratory arrest. Prehospital: As above.
Dextromethorphan (cough syrup/cold medications)	Mild: Restlessness and euphoria and signs of intoxication. Moderate: Slurred speech, lack of coordination, memory loss, hallucinations, and "stoned" appearance. Severe: Altered state of consciousness, impaired vision, hearing, emotional detachment, inability to comprehend spoken words, leading to hallucinations, delusions, tachycardia, temporary blindness, and respiratory arrest. Some people exhibit violent or psychotic behavior. Prehospital: As above; restrain if necessary.

Cardiac	Digitalis (digoxin) toxicity may cause (initially) increasing fatigue, lethargy, depression, nausea, "halo" vision, and vomiting progressing to sudden changes in heart rhythm, such as an irregular rhythm, palpitations, heart block, tachycardia, and, later, bradycardia. Prehospital: Manage the patient's airway/ventilation/oxygen supplementation and circulation as needed.
Psychiatric	Benzodiazepine toxicity may result from accidental or intentional overdose with such drugs as Xanax and Valium. Indications are often nonspecific neurological changes such as lethargy, dizziness, alterations in consciousness, and ataxia. Respiratory depression and hypotension are rare complications. Prehospital: Provide supportive care. Mild lithium toxicity (Eskalith, Lithobid) can include severe vomiting and diarrhea, increased muscle tremors and twitching, lethargy, body aches, ataxia, ringing in the ears, blurry vision, vertigo, or hyperactive deep-tendon reflexes. More severe symptoms can include elevated temperature, low urine output, hypotension, heart abnormalities, decreased level of consciousness, seizures, coma, or death. Prehospital: Manage the patient's airway/ventilation/oxygen supplementation and circulation as needed.

Narcotics

Narcotics include opiates (drugs derived from opium) and opioids (synthetic narcotics). Drugs frequently abused include heroin and many prescription drugs such as morphine, meperidine, fentanyl (pills and patches), oxycodone, hydrocodone, buprenorphine, and methadone. Patients often crush pills and snort or inject them to increase the effects. Because tolerance to the drugs occurs, patients tend to take higher and higher doses, resulting in addiction and an increasing risk of overdose. Narcotics reduce pain and provide a feeling of euphoria or well-being as well as drowsiness. Symptoms of overdose may include slurred speech, pupil (pinpoint) constriction, nausea, hypotension, vomiting, lack of coordination, alterations of consciousness, coma, respiratory depression, cyanosis, and cardiac arrest (death). Patients may have a runny, irritated nose from snorting drugs or may have needle marks from injecting. Prehospital: Manage the patient's airway/ventilation/oxygen supplementation, and provide CPR if necessary. Administer naloxone (an opioid reversal agent) per autoinjector or nasal spray if protocol allows.

Spontaneous Pneumothorax

Spontaneous pneumothorax is air in the pleural space that causes the lung to collapse but without an obvious cause. Symptoms include an abrupt onset of sharp chest pain on the affected side, dyspnea, difficulty breathing, and decreased/absent respirations on the affected side.

- Primary (no underlying lung disease): It is most common in tall, thin adolescents and young adults and is associated with cigarette smoking. Often resolves without treatment and rarely progresses to tension pneumothorax.
- Secondary (underlying lung disease): It is most common in those with chronic obstructive pulmonary disease (COPD), cystic fibrosis, and severe asthma, and it poses a risk of death because of respiratory compromise. Patients may develop hypoxemia, altered mental status, coma, and tension pneumothorax.

Prehospital: Manage the patient's airway/ventilation/oxygen supplementation, place the patient in a position of comfort, and transport. A large spontaneous pneumothorax will require catheter aspiration of air or insertion of a chest tube.

Epiglottitis

Acute epiglottitis (supraglottitis) occurs in children primarily from 1 to 8 years old and in young adults. Acute epiglottitis requires immediate medical attention because it can rapidly become obstructive. The onset is usually very sudden and often occurs during the night. The patient may awaken suddenly with a fever, but he or she usually does not have a cough. Symptoms include:

- Tripod position: Sits upright, leaning forward, mouth open, and tongue protruding.
- Agitation: Appears restless, tense, and agitated.
- Drooling: Excess secretions combined with pain or dysphagia and a mouth-open position.
- Voice: No hoarseness, but his or her voice sounds thick and "froglike."
- Cyanosis: Color is usually pale and sallow initially but may progress to frank cyanosis.
- Throat: On examination, the epiglottis appears bright red and swollen. Note: The patient's throat should not be examined with a tongue blade unless intubation and tracheostomy equipment is immediately available because the examination can trigger an obstruction.

Prehospital: Provide rapid transport, administer high-flow oxygen with blow-by mask, or provide slow ventilation with a BVM.

Respiratory Conditions

Respiratory condition	Assessment/Findings	Prehospital
Asthma	An immune response causes constriction of bronchi and inflammation and increased secretions in the lower airways. Symptoms include cough, wheezing, diminished breath sounds, and dyspnea.	Assist with albuterol (nebulized/metered dose) and oxygen (6–8 LPM), and provide airway management/ventilation. Provide CPAP for moderate/severe cases. Severe: Provide rapid transport.
Pulmonary edema	Often secondary to congestive heart failure or pulmonary embolus, fluid collects in the lung alveoli (air sacs), resulting in severe shortness of breath, wheezing, rapid pulse, cough, and chest pain.	Place the patient in a position of comfort (usually with head elevated), manage the patient's airway/ventilation, and provide supplemental oxygen. Severe: Provide rapid transport.
Pneumonia	Infection of the lungs (bacterial, viral, fungal, or parasitic) resulting in fever, chills, cough, purulent sputum, and difficulty breathing, chest pain on cough or deep inhalation, and headache. Infants may exhibit sternal retraction, decreased feeding, and irritability. Adolescents may have vomiting, diarrhea, sore throat, and ache along with typical symptoms.	Use standard and droplet precautions, including wearing a protective face mask. Place the patient in a position of comfort (usually with the head elevated), and manage the patient's airway/ventilation/oxygen supplementation. Severe: Provide rapid transport.

Pertussis (whooping cough)	Severe persistent "whooping" cough, thick sputum, postcough emesis, petechiae on the upper body, and sclera from exertion. Infants may develop CNS damage, apnea, or pneumonia; children may develop hernia or muscle damage; and adults may develop hernia or a fractured rib.	Use standard and droplet precautions, provide the patient a position of comfort, and manage the patient's airway/ventilation/oxygen supplementation as needed.
Cystic fibrosis	Progressive congenital disease that particularly affects the pancreas and lungs, causing the production of thick mucus that clogs the lungs and causes recurrent bacterial infections. Symptoms include severe cough, sputum, fever, and dyspnea.	Use standard and droplet precautions, and provide the patient a position of comfort. Manage the patient's airway/ventilation/oxygen supplementation. Severe: Provide rapid transport.
Chronic obstructive pulmonary disease (COPD)	Disease with limitations of airflow, narrowing airways, exertional dyspnea, chronic cough, right-sided heart failure (cor pulmonale), damaged, distended alveoli, and barrel chest. Symptoms include severe dyspnea, cough, and the tripod position.	Manage the patient's airway/ventilation, and provide oxygen per nonrebreather mask to maintain oxygen saturation >90%. Provide the patient a position of comfort. Severe: Provide rapid transport.

Metered-Dose Inhaler (MIDI/MDI) and the Small-Volume Nebulizer

The EMT may assist the patient with use of a metered-dose inhaler (MIDI/MDI) or a small-volume nebulizer for medications such as albuterol, according to protocol as follows:

- The **MIDI/MDI** is a pressurized cartridge that is used for administration of a specific dose of an aerosolized medication. Shake the medication vigorously before use, prime if it is the initial use, position 4 cm (two finger widths) away from the patient's mouth or between the lips, have the patient exhale and breathe in slowly and completely while the MIDI is activated, and then have the patient hold the breath for 10 seconds, waiting 1 minute between puffs. Stop the treatment if the patient becomes shaky, dizzy, coughs uncontrollably, has palpitations, or has a pulse increase of ≥20 bpm. Resume slowly after 5 to 10 minutes.
- A **small-volume nebulizer** includes a nebulizer cup that holds 2 to 4 mL of medication, air tubing, a compressor to aerosolize the medication, and a T-piece and mouthpiece or face mask for delivery. Dilute the medication with sterile NS or water, not tap water, if necessary. Have the patient sit upright for treatment, breathing normally through the mouth and using the mouthpiece or face mask.

Sickle Cell Disease

Sickle cell disease is a recessive genetic disorder of chromosome 11, causing hemoglobin to be defective so that the red blood cells (RBCs) are sickle-shaped and inflexible, resulting in their accumulating in small vessels and causing painful blockages. Although normal RBCs survive for 120 days, sickled blood cells may survive only 10–20 days, stressing the bone marrow that can't produce RBCs fast enough and resulting in anemia. Different types of **crises** occur (aplastic, hemolytic, vaso-occlusive, and sequestering), which can cause infarctions in organs, severe pain, damage to organs, and rapid enlargement of the liver and spleen. Vaso-occlusive crisis is common in adolescents and adults, and it can be triggered by sickness, stress, dehydration, temperature changes, and high altitude. Young children are prone to splenic sequestration (RBCs trapped in the spleen, causing it to enlarge and sometimes rupture), which is characterized by pain in the left abdomen. Prehospital: Manage the patient's airway/ventilation/oxygen supplementation and circulation, provide emotional support, and provide rapid transport for severe symptoms.

Clotting Disorders

Clotting disorders include the following:

- <u>Hemophilia</u> is an inherited disorder in which the person lacks adequate clotting factors, which results in bleeding with trauma, bruising, spontaneous hemorrhage (often in the joints), and epistaxis. There are three primary types: A (80%–90%), B, and C.
- <u>Disseminated intravascular coagulation (DIC)</u> (consumption coagulopathy) is a secondary disorder that is triggered by another event, such as trauma, congenital heart disease, necrotizing enterocolitis, sepsis, and severe viral infections. DIC triggers coagulation (clotting) and hemorrhage through a complex series of events, with clotting and hemorrhage occurring simultaneously, putting the patient at risk of death.
- <u>Von Willebrand's disease</u> is a group of congenital bleeding disorders (inherited from either parent) affecting 1%–2% of the population, associated with deficiency or lack of von Willebrand factor (vWF), a glycoprotein.

Prehospital: Monitor for signs of bleeding, and manage the patient's airway/ventilation/oxygen supplementation. Provide rapid transport for hemorrhage or acute blood loss resulting in hypotension.

Hemodialysis

Hemodialysis is used primarily for those who have progressed from renal insufficiency to uremia with end-stage renal (kidney) disease (ESRD). With hemodialysis, blood is circulated outside of the body through a dialyzer (a synthetic semipermeable membrane), which filters the blood and removes waste products and excess fluids. A vascular access device, such as a catheter, fistula, or graft must be established for hemodialysis with fistulas and grafts usually being placed in an arm and a catheter being placed in the upper chest (into the superior vena cava). Tubing from the dialysis machine attaches to the access device for treatments, which are usually done for 4 hours three times weekly. Emergent conditions include low BP, nausea/vomiting, irregular pulse, cardiac arrest, bleeding from the access site, and difficulty breathing. Missed treatments may result in electrolyte excess, weakness, and pulmonary edema. Prehospital: Manage the patient's airway/ventilation/oxygen supplementation, apply pressure to stop any bleeding, position the patie͛ flat if he or she is in shock, and position him or her upright if having difficulty breathing.

ʾDialysis

ʾlysis is used to remove waste products and excess fluids from those with ESRD. A
ʾ into the peritoneal cavity of the abdomen. The peritoneum comprises the visceral
ʾing of the gut and other viscera), which makes up about 80% of the total
ʾa, and the parietal perineum (lining the abdominal cavity), which is the most
ʾl dialysis. A dialysate solution is instilled (usually about 2 L for adults but
ʾbout 10 minutes) through the catheter, the catheter is clamped, and the

solution (dwell) is left in place for 3–6 hours. The solution is then drained (usually for about 20 minutes), and the process is repeated with new dialysate. Peritoneal dialysis increases the risk of obesity, peritonitis, hernia, malnutrition, hypertriglyceridemia, and back pain. Obesity, older adulthood, and lack of social support are contraindications for peritoneal dialysis. Prehospital: Manage the patient's airway/ventilation/oxygen supplementation, use contact precautions if there is purulent drainage from catheter site, and position the patient for comfort.

Urinary Catheter Management

A **urinary catheter** is inserted through the urethra and into the bladder to drain urine. Straight catheterizations are done with sterile catheters periodically to empty the bladder or to relieve urinary retention, whereas retention catheters (Foley) have a balloon that inflates to keep the catheter in place for continuous drainage. Foley catheters may be indicated for patients with neuromuscular disorders, incontinence, urinary retention, dementia, or urinary disorders. Catheters may also be inserted suprapubically (above the pubis bone) directly into the bladder, especially for males with long-term catheterization. Urinary collection bags should be kept below the level of the bladder, and the tubing is secured so that the catheter is not inadvertently pulled out, causing trauma to the urethra, especially in males. Thick, cloudy urine may indicate infection. Scant urine and lower abdominal pain/distension may indicate blockage of the catheter. Milking the catheter may help relieve a blockage. When removing a Foley catheter, the balloon must first be deflated. Prehospital: Provide supportive care.

Vaginal Bleeding

Vaginal bleeding may indicate heavy menstrual bleeding (menorrhagia) or abnormal bleeding between cycles (metrorrhagia). Vaginal bleeding may also be an indication of an ectopic pregnancy or spontaneous abortion; in postmenopausal women, it may be a sign of endometrial cancer. Menorrhagia may result from hormonal imbalance, clotting disorders, uterine fibroids, and endometrial polyps. Metrorrhagia may result from infection, cancer, and cervical/endometrial polyps. Symptoms may include cramping and abdominal pain, depending on the cause. It's important to determine when the bleeding started and about how much blood had been lost (the number of sanitary pads that are saturated per hour, for example) as well as the presence or absence of pain. If blood loss is excessive, the patient may exhibit signs of shock. Prehospital: Use standard precautions, manage the patient's airway/ventilation/oxygen supplementation. Monitor vital signs. Position the patient flat for shock, and provide IV access and fluids.

Female Reproductive System

The **female reproductive system** includes the ovaries, fallopian tubes, uterus, cervix, vagina, vulva, labia minora, labia majora, clitoris, and breasts. Functions include ovulation, fertilization, menstruation, pregnancy, and lactation. Menarche (onset of menses) is usually between 9 and 15, but it may occur in younger girls and should be considered as a possibility with younger girls. Menopause occurs at approximately age 50, usually following a period of about 10 years of irregular periods during which time the person may become pregnant. The normal menstrual cycle is 28 days, but it may be up to 45 days in adolescents. Assessment should include abdominal or vaginal pain, vaginal bleeding or discharge, fever, nausea and vomiting, and dizziness. Patients should have their privacy protected during an examination, and the EMT should communicate openly, asking for permission to touch the patient. The EMT should consider the possibility of pregnancy or sexually transmitted disease with any abnormal condition.

Sexual Assault

The crime scenes associated with a **sexual assault** include the patient (body, injuries, clothing, and emotional response) and the place the assault occurred. A victim of sexual assault has the right to consent to or refuse each element of a sexual assault evaluation, although some states may mandate reporting of sexual assault to the authorities. The EMT should wear disposable gloves when handling clothing, and clothing should be handled gently so that evidence, such as strands of hair or other materials, is not lost in transfer. Documenting the assault should be done in detail with direct quotations. If the patient refuses transport, the best approach is to point out services that could benefit the patient, such as prophylaxis to prevent STDs and pregnancy. Patients are often frightened and confused, so pressuring them to protect others or trying to frighten them more by suggesting that they might be pregnant or develop an STD is a negative approach that may backfire.

Sexually Transmitted Diseases

Disease	Characteristics/Considerations
Gonorrhea	Caused by the bacterial species *Neisseria gonorrhoeae*. Transmission is through anal, oral, or vaginal sex. The incubation period is 3 to 8 days. Male symptoms include painful urination, purulent discharge from the penis, and swollen testicles. Females are asymptomatic, or they may have mild difficulty urinating. Complications include prostatitis, orchitis, epididymitis, and sterility (males) and pelvic inflammatory disease and disseminated disease (females). It is treated with antibiotics. The infection may pass to a newborn during birth, causing gonorrheal eye infection and blindness unless eye prophylaxis is provided. Prehospital: Use standard precautions.
Chlamydia	Caused by the bacterial species *Chlamydia trachomatis*. Transmission is through anal, oral, or vaginal sex. It often occurs with gonorrhea. Symptoms: Many are asymptomatic, but the disease can spread and cause urethritis, proctitis, and epididymitis (males) and painful intercourse, pelvic inflammatory disease, fallopian tube damage, and vaginal bleeding (females). Complications include sterility and infertility. Treatment is with antibiotics. Prehospital: Use standard precautions.
Syphilis (*Treponema pallidum*)	Bacterial infection transmitted through oral, anal, or vaginal sex and needle sharing. The incubation period is 10 to 90 days. <u>Primary symptoms</u> (3–8 weeks): Chancres (very contagious). <u>Secondary symptoms</u> (1–2 years): Flu-like symptoms and rash, weight loss, and hair loss. <u>Latent symptoms</u> (>2 years): Asymptomatic. Noncontagious after 4 years. Treatment is antibiotics. <u>Late/Tertiary symptoms:</u> Gummas (lesions) in multiple organs, heart abnormalities, CNS impairment with psychosis, confusion, ataxia, and difficulty speaking. Prehospital: Standard precautions.
Genital herpes (herpes simplex virus 2)	Transmitted though oral, anal, or vaginal sex. The virus enters nerve endings, travels to the nerve ganglion, and stays dormant until reactivated by stress, immunosuppression, menstruation, sunburn, illness, or other triggers. Initial symptoms: Small vesicular lesions in genital area that rupture and leave open crusting sores; painful urination; flu-like symptoms. Recurrent symptoms are less severe, lasting 8–12 days. Complications include dissemination to other areas of the body, aseptic meningitis, and damage to nerves resulting in atonic bladder, constipation, and impotence. Treatment is with antiviral agents. Prehospital: Use standard, contact, and airborne precautions until disseminated herpes is ruled out.

Musculoskeletal System

The **musculoskeletal system** includes 203 bones including long bones (e.g., the femur in the thigh), short bones (e.g., the carpal bones in the fingers), and flat bones (e.g., the sternum). The outer hard shell of the bone is the cortex, and the inner porous area is the trabecular bone. The vertebrae lack the cortex layer. Long bones have three parts: The middle section is the diaphysis, followed by the metaphyses, and then the epiphyses (the bone ends). In growing children, an epiphyseal plate of cartilage separates the metaphyses and epiphyses, allowing bone growth. This closes in adults, but damage to this area in a child may impair bone growth. The middle part of the short bones contains yellow bone marrow (fatty tissue). Red bone marrow, which produces blood cells, is found in the middle of the flat bones (pelvis, sternum, ribs, and scapula) and at the ends (epiphyses) of long bones. The skeletal system is connected by cartilage and tendons, and it is protected, supported, and allowed movement by about 700 soft-tissue muscles.

Nontraumatic Fractures

Nontraumatic fractures occur when the bone weakens and can no longer support the body, such as may occur with a cancerous tumor of the bone or osteoporosis. Common fractures associated with osteoporosis include fractures of the vertebrae and hip. Osteoporotic fractures are most common in older adults, but they may also occur in adolescents with eating disorders. Infants and young children with multiple nontraumatic, nonabusive fractures may have a genetic disorder, such as osteogenesis imperfecta. Assessment of suspected fractures includes evaluating pain/tenderness, swelling around the fracture site, loss of sensation or movement, circulatory impairment (note the color of the skin, pallor or cyanosis), and deformity (especially noticeable in limb fractures). Prehospital: Splint extremity fractures; manage the patient's airway/ventilation/oxygen supplementation as needed; and provide transport for treatment.

Nosebleed (Epistaxis)

Recurrent **nosebleed (epistaxis)** is common in young children (2–10), especially boys, and it is often related to nose picking, dry climate, trauma, or central heating. Incidence also increases between 50–80 years of age and may be associated with nonsteroidal anti-inflammatory drugs (NSAIDs), hypertension, and anticoagulants. Patients abusing cocaine may suffer nosebleeds because of damage to the mucosa. The anterior (front) nares have plentiful blood vessels and bleed easily, usually from one nostril. Bleeding in the posterior (back) nares is more dangerous and can result in considerable blood loss. Blood may flow through both nostrils or backward into the throat, and the person may be observed swallowing and may vomit blood. The blood may block the airway in unconscious patients. Prehospital: Sit the patient in an upright position, leaning forward so the blood doesn't flow down the throat if the patient is conscious; pinch nostrils together firmly for at least 10 minutes; and advise the patient to avoid sniffing or blowing the nose.

Shock and Resuscitation

Shock

Shock is a life-threatening condition that occurs when the tissues do not receive adequate oxygen, such as with severe bleeding or fluid loss, severe infection, heart failure, or abnormal dilation of the blood vessels. Signs/Symptoms of shock include the following: extreme thirst; anxiety and restlessness; weak, rapid pulse; altered mental status progressing to loss of consciousness; rapid, shallow respirations; hypotension (low BP—often a late sign); and cool, clammy, pale skin with mottling sometimes on extremities from inadequate perfusion. If left untreated, shock may lead to cardiac arrest. Note that geriatric patients may have a higher baseline respiration and heart rate and irregular pulse. Prehospital: Request the assistance of advanced EMS if necessary, apply pressure to control the bleeding, perform spinal stabilization if needed, place the patient in the shock position (flat with feet elevated above the level of the heart, 8 to 12 inches), manage the patient's airway/ventilation and administer high-concentration oxygen, provide warming blankets to maintain body temperature, and provide reassurance. Provide rapid transport if needed. **Shock** generally occurs in stages as the body tries to compensate: Compensated shock occurs in the early stage while the body speeds up the heart rate and respirations and diverts blood to the vital organs (resulting in pale, cool skin) to maintain adequate perfusion and BP. Decompensated shock occurs when the body can no longer compensate and the BP falls and symptoms worsen. With irreversible shock, recovery is no longer possible because of cell damage caused by inadequate oxygenation and perfusion. Types of shock include the following:

Type of shock	Cause
Cardiogenic	Heart failure, myocardial infarction, drug overdose, dysrhythmia, congenital heart disease.
Distributive	Anaphylaxis, drug overdose.
Hypovolemic	Hemorrhage, severe vomiting and/or diarrhea, severe burns, dehydration.
Obstructive	Pneumothorax, pericardial tamponade.
Neurogenic	Spinal cord injury (a form of distributive shock because of decreased vascular tone).
Septic	Sepsis, severe infections. (This is also a form of distributive shock.)

Signs and symptoms are similar for all types of shock even though the mechanisms are different.

Respiratory Failure/Arrest

Respiratory failure occurs when ventilation is insufficient for adequate gas exchange so that levels of carbon dioxide in the blood increase and levels of oxygen decrease. Respiratory failure may result from respiratory infection (pneumonia, tuberculosis), heart failure, chronic respiratory illness (asthma, chronic bronchitis, COPD), trauma, and depression of the central nervous system (usually from medications or trauma). Respiratory failure may be acute with sudden onset or chronic, developing over time. If untreated, respiratory failure can lead to **respiratory arrest**, which in turn leads to cardiac arrest. Indications of respiratory failure include altered mental status, cyanosis, labored breathing (dyspnea and orthopnea), coughing, fatigue, diminished breath sounds, and the presence of rales (crackles) and rhonchi (snoring/whistling sound). Patients may have hemoptysis (bloody sputum). The patient's oxygen saturation level is lower than 90% per pulse oximeter. Prehospital: Manage the patient's airway/ventilation/oxygen supplementation; positive-pressure ventilation may be needed. Place the patient in a position of comfort (usually high Fowler's).

Cardiopulmonary Resuscitation (CPR) for Cardiac Arrest

Cardiac arrest of unknown cause in adults or children is usually treated as though it were ventricular fibrillation or pulseless ventricular tachycardia, but the protocol varies. **Cardiopulmonary resuscitation (CPR)** involves the following components:

- Immediate defibrillation (one shock) is performed according to protocol with an AED/manual defibrillator (preferred) followed by CPR, beginning with compressions (30:2 compression to ventilation at the rate of 100–120 per minute at least 2 inches deep; two-finger compressions, to one-third of the chest depth for infants and children) for 2 minutes/five cycles and repeat defibrillation.
- Repeat cycles of 2 minutes CPR and defibrillation. (Laypeople may use compression-only CPR.)
- If a defibrillator is not readily available, CPR may begin first. Note that if a BVM is used, the break in compressions should not exceed 10 seconds. If an advanced airway/intubation is in place, ventilation should be at the rate of 8 to 10 per minute, maintaining oxygen saturation $\geq 94\%$ but $<100\%$ with ventilation between compressions.
- The $ETCO_2$ value should be 10–20 mm Hg if chest compressions are adequate, increasing to 35 to 45 mm Hg with the return of spontaneous circulation (ROSC).

Ethical Issues in Withholding Resuscitation Attempts

Although the goal of EMS is to save lives, it is not always possible or ethical to carry out resuscitation efforts. **Withholding resuscitation** is justified under the following conditions:

- The patient's condition is not compatible with life (massive injuries, decapitation, crushed chest, severe open head injury with loss of brain tissue), and the patient is not breathing and has no pulse.
- The patient exhibits obvious signs of death, such as rigor mortis or livor mortis, indicating that he or she can no longer be resuscitated.
- The patient has a do-not-resuscitate (DNR) form available, and it is properly signed. Note: The EMT cannot accept the word of family or friends that the patient does not want to be resuscitated without a DNR order.
- Conditions are unsafe to approach the patient and/or administer resuscitation efforts. This may occur, for example, if there are gunshots heard in the area, if the patient is pinned under a motor vehicle, or if the patient cannot safely be reached in time because of difficult terrain.

Heimlich Maneuver

The universal sign of choking is when a person clutches his or her throat and appears to be choking or gasping for breath. If the person can speak ("Can you speak?") or cough, the **Heimlich maneuver** is not usually necessary. The Heimlich maneuver can be done with the victim sitting, standing, or supine. The Heimlich procedure for children (≥ 1 year) and adults is as follows:

- Wrap your arms around the victim's waist from the back if sitting or standing. Make a fist and place the thumb side against the victim's abdomen slightly above the umbilicus. Grasp this hand with the other and thrust sharply upward to force air out of the lungs.
- Repeat as needed.

- If the victim loses consciousness, ease him or her into a supine position on the floor, place your hands similarly to CPR but over the abdomen while sitting astride the victim's legs. Repeat upward compressions five times. If no ventilation occurs, attempt to sweep the mouth and ventilate the lungs mouth to mouth. Repeat compressions and ventilations until recovery.

Indications of choking in infants of less than 1 year include lack of breathing, gasping, cyanosis, and the inability to cry. The procedure for **Heimlich chest thrusts** includes the following:

- Position the infant in the prone (face-down) position along your forearm with the infant's head being lower than the trunk, being sure to support the head so the airway is not blocked.
- Using the heel of the hand, deliver five forceful upward blows between the shoulder blades.
- Sandwich the child between your two arms, and turn the infant into the supine position and drape over your thigh with his or her head lower than the trunk and the head supported.
- Using two fingers (as for CPR compressions), give up to five thrusts (about 1.5 inches deep) to the lower third of the sternum.
- Only do a finger sweep and remove a foreign object if the object is visible. Repeat five back blows, five chest thrusts until the foreign body is ejected.
- If the infant loses consciousness, begin CPR. If a pulse is noted but spontaneous respirations are absent, continue with ventilation only.

Emergency Defibrillation with an Automated External Defibrillator (AED)

Emergency defibrillation is done for acute ventricular fibrillation or ventricular tachycardia with no audible or palpable pulse; it is ineffective for asystole or pulseless electrical activity. Defibrillation delivers an electrical discharge through paddles applied to both sides of the chest. **Automated external defibrillators (AEDs)** are frequently used by first responders, although manual defibrillators require less downtime from CPR. The procedure is as follows:

- Turn on the AED.
- Apply pads to the chest (the position may vary according to the manufacturer). Infants and small children: If the pads may touch, apply one to the chest and one to the back.
- Plug in the connector if necessary.
- Do not touch the patient while the AED analyzes the heart rhythm.
- Follow the directions for shocking, and warn others to stand clear.
- Continue CPR, beginning with compressions for 2 minutes/five cycles between defibrillations.
- If the patient is wet, wipe off his or her chest before applying the pads. Remove any transdermal patches on the chest, and shave excessive hair before applying the pads. If the patient has an implanted device, the pads should be placed at least 1 inch (2.5 cm) away.

Trauma

Blunt Trauma (Nonbleeding)

Motor vehicle crashes	Result in 30%–40% of accidental deaths and half of closed-head and spinal cord injuries with injuries usually more serious with ejection, lateral (T-bone) impacts, and unrestrained patients, although lap belts increase the risk of abdominal injury (bowel injury in children). Shoulder belts may cause vascular injuries. Injuries include crush (compression), shear (tearing), and burst (rupture from sudden increase in pressure). Risk of death increases if another vehicle occupant dies. Most frontal collisions result in injuries from impact with the steering wheel, dashboard, windshield, or floorboards. More severe injuries occur at speeds of >25 mph.
Motorcycle crashes	75% of deaths are from head injuries, but injuries to the spine, pelvis, and extremities, including limb loss, are common.
Pedestrian/ Motor vehicle impacts	Often results in Waddell's triad (tibiofibular or femur fracture, trunk injury, and head/face injury). Small children are often run over, and adults are thrown over the car by the impact. Intra-abdominal injuries and pelvic fractures may occur from fender contact with the hips.
Falls	The most common cause of accidental death in geriatric patients is by falling. Anticoagulants increase the risk of injury with falls. The degree of injury depends on patient's weight and fall distance. Injuries are most severe with a fall distance of >20 feet for adults and >10 feet for children. A three-story fall results in 50% mortality; the mortality is almost 100% for five-story falls. Horizontal landings cause fewer injuries (hand, wrist, head/face, and abdominal) than feet-first landings, which often result in fractures of the heel, leg, pelvis, and/or vertebrae.
Sports injuries/ Play	Injuries vary depending on the type of injury but can include head injuries, musculoskeletal injuries, and abdominal injuries. Helmet or knee contact to the flank area may cause kidney injury. The most common injuries are strains, sprains, and knee injuries.
Assaults	Assaults are most common in young males and include facial and head injuries. Severe torso injuries may occur with kicking/stomping. If the patient is intoxicated and has altered consciousness, the patient is treated as having a head injury. Assaults include domestic violence and child abuse, with distinctive patterns of injury.

Penetrating Trauma (Bleeding)

Gunshot wounds	Solid organs (brain, liver, spleen) often suffer more damage than more elastic tissues (fat, lungs). If a bullet is not deformed after entering the tissue, it tends to tumble (180°), creating a tunnel of injury (permanent cavity) and damage to the surrounding tissue (temporary cavity). If the bullet is deformed, it causes more severe localized tissue damage. Bullets usually have a straight trajectory, but they may be deflected if they strike bone. Shotgun blasts within 15 feet cause more damage than other gunshot wounds, but they are usually less severe at a distance.
Stab wounds	<u>Stab:</u> Includes hand-driven objects (knives, glass shards, ice picks, or pieces of metal/wood). Surface puncture wounds are often small, but their depth varies according to the instrument used, which should be removed surgically. <u>Slash:</u> These are usually long but not deep lacerations. <u>Impalement:</u> This usually results from objects larger than a knife, often from a fall onto an object, but it can include arrows and nails from pneumatic tools.

Revised Trauma Score (RTS)and Primary Assessment

The **revised trauma score (RTS)** uses the Glasgow Coma Scale (GCS) score, systolic blood pressure (BP), and respiration rate to establish a score for triage (START). Scores may range from 0 to 12. For triage purposes, an RTS of 12 indicates delayed treatment, 11 indicates urgent, and a score of 3 to 10 indicates that immediate treatment is required. Scores less than 3 indicate death. However, the scores are weighted differently, with the GCS score having the greatest weight (RTS = 0.9368 GCS + 0.7326 BP + 0.2908 R), so a reference chart must be used to determine the actual score based on the initial assessment of the patient. **Primary assessment** of trauma patients should include evaluation of the airway, breathing, and circulation (including observing for deviated septum, changes in chest wall motion, fractures, sucking chest wounds, crepitation [of the neck and chest] from air) as well as an assessment of disability with a brief neurological exam (pupils, limb movement) and GSC/RTS. Removing the patient's clothing for examination and logrolling him or her are part of the assessment.

GCS (score)	Systolic BP (score)	Respirations (score)
13-15 (4)	>89 (4)	10-29 (4)
9-12 (3)	76-89 (3)	>29 (3)
6-8 (2)	50-75 (2)	6-9 (2)
4-5 (1)	1-49 (1)	1-5 (1)
3 (0)	0 (0)	0(0)

Types of Bleeding

Types of bleeding	Characteristics
Arterial	Bright-red spurting blood that is difficult to control; it lessens as the BP falls.
Venous	Dark-red blood flowing in a steady stream; it, may be copious, but it is easier to control than an arterial bleed.
Capillary	Oozing; it usually clots spontaneously.
Internal	Usually evidenced by increasing signs of shock and/or discolored swollen, painful tissue, guarding, coughing up blood, or rectal bleeding. Long-bone fractures (femur) and pelvic fractures may result in severe blood loss.

Prehospital

Using standard precautions and PPE as indicated, apply sterile gauze dressing and pressure with the fingertips if it is a small bleed or apply direct hand pressure if it is more copious. As dressings saturate, add new dressings but don't remove the old ones. A tourniquet may be needed if bleeding is uncontrolled. Maintain the patient in the shock position, especially with an arterial bleed or severe blood loss, and keep him or her warm. Avoid giving food or fluids and transport immediately for severe bleeding. Severity relates to the rate of blood loss volume and the age and health of the patient. The blood volume is less with pediatric patients. Moving the injured area, a change in body temperature, medications, and the removal of bandages may impair clotting.

Chest Wounds

Type	Characteristics	Prehospital
Sucking	This is an open pneumothorax in which air sucks into the thoracic cavity, deflating the lung, usually through a penny-size or larger wound. Patients will exhibit respiratory distress, absent breath sounds on the affected side, wound gurgling on inspiration, and bubbling of blood around the wound.	Apply an occlusive dressing with an Asherman Chest Seal dressing or with Vaseline gauze covered with secured (taped on three sides) plastic wrap or aluminum foil and place the patient in position of comfort.
Impalement	This is a penetrating wound with an object impaled into the chest. Symptoms may be similar to those listed above, depending on the site of impalement and the depth. Impalement may cause hemothorax, tension pneumothorax, or pericardial tamponade.	Expose the wound area, and secure the object manually with a bulky dressing. Do not remove the object unless it is necessary for performing chest compressions (CPR). Control the bleeding.

Blunt Cardiac Trauma

Blunt cardiac trauma most often occurs as the result of motor vehicle accidents, falls, or other blows to the chest, which can result in respiratory distress as well as hypovolemia from rupture of the great vessels of the heart and/or cardiac failure from cardiac tamponade or increasing intrathoracic pressure. The heart is particularly vulnerable to chest trauma, with the right atrium and right ventricle being the most commonly injured because they are anterior to the rest of the heart. *Commotio cordis*, an often-lethal dysrhythmia from a blow to the pericardial area, may occur (most common in young males with sports injuries). Cardiac trauma may be difficult to identify because of other injuries, but if it is suspected, an ECG should be done and any abnormalities (dysrhythmias, ST changes, sinus tachycardia, or heart block) should be noted. Decreased cardiac output and cerebral oxygenation may result in severe agitation with combative behavior. Prehospital: Provide CPR and defibrillation if indicated; manage the patient's airway/ventilation/oxygen supplementation; provide an IV access line with severe injury; monitor changes in the patient's level of consciousness.

Jugular Venous Pressure

Jugular venous pressure (neck vein) is used to assess the cardiac output and pressure in the right heart because the pulsations relate to changes in pressure in the right atrium. This procedure is usually not accurate if the pulse rate is >100. This is a noninvasive estimation of the central venous pressure and waveform. Measurement should be done with the internal jugular if possible; otherwise, the external jugular may be used.

- Elevate the patient's head to 45° (and to 90° if necessary) with the patient's head turned to the opposite side of examination.
- Position the light at an angle to illuminate the veins and shadows.
- Measure the height of the jugular vein pulsation above the sternal joint, using a ruler.
- The normal height of the jugular vein pulsation is ≤4 cm above the sternal angle.

Increased height (>4 cm) indicates increased pressure in the right atrium and right heart failure. It may also indicate pericarditis or tricuspid stenosis. Laughing or coughing may trigger the Valsalva response and also cause a pressure increase.

Fractured Ribs and Flail Chest

Fractured ribs usually result from severe blunt trauma (motor vehicle accident, physical abuse). Underlying injuries should be expected according to the area of fractures as follows:

- Upper two ribs: Injuries to trachea, bronchi, or great vessels.
- Right-sided ≥ rib 8: Liver trauma.
- Left-sided ≥ rib 8: Spleen trauma.

Pain may be the primary symptom of rib fractures, resulting in shallow breathing. **Flail chest** (more common in adults and adolescents than children) occurs when at least three adjacent ribs are fractured, anteriorly and posteriorly, so that they float free of the rib cage. Variations include the sternum floating with ribs fractured on both sides. With flail chest, the chest wall cannot support changes in intrathoracic pressure, so paradoxical respirations occur with the flail area contracting on inspiration and expanding on expiration. Ventilation decreases. Prehospital: Manage the patient's airway/ventilation/oxygen supplementation (PPV with BVM or intubation), provide cardiac monitoring and supportive care, and observe for signs of tension pneumothorax or hemothorax.

Hemothorax

Hemothorax occurs with bleeding into the pleural space, usually from major vascular injury such as tears in intercostal vessels, lacerations of great vessels, or trauma to lung tissue. It is most common with penetrating wounds. A small bleed may be self-limiting and seal, but a tear in a large vessel can result in massive bleeding, followed quickly by hypovolemic shock from decreased circulating blood. The pressure from the blood may result in the inability of the lung to ventilate and a mediastinal shift. Clots in the chest area may trigger fibrinolysis, which breaks down clots and increases bleeding. Often a hemothorax occurs with a pneumothorax, especially in severe chest trauma. Further symptoms include severe respiratory distress, decreased breath sounds, unequal breath sounds, dullness on auscultation, jugular venous distension, and shock. Prehospital: Manage the patient's airway/ventilation/oxygen supplementation, request assistance for an IV access line and fluid bolus for shock but avoid aggressive fluids because of the risk of hemodilution, provide the patient a position of comfort (the shock position if necessary), and provide rapid transport.

Tension Pneumothorax

If not treated promptly, a sucking chest wound (open pneumothorax) may progress to a **tension pneumothorax,** especially if mechanical ventilation is used. A tension pneumothorax occurs when pressure in the pleural space exceeds that of the atmosphere, causing a mediastinal shift (which is usually difficult to assess visually) with displacement of the trachea away from the affected site, putting pressure against the great vessels (decreasing cardiac output) and putting pressure against the heart (resulting in tachycardia). Patients are usually in severe respiratory distress with jugular vein distension, absent breath sounds on the affected side, narrow pulse pressure, pulsus paradoxus, and unequal chest rise. Prehospital: Place an airtight seal or an Asherman Chest Seal over the open wound, manage the patient's airway/ventilation/oxygen supplementation to an oxygen saturation level of ≥94%, provide cardiac monitoring, request assistance for an IV access line, and provide rapid transport. Tension pneumothorax will require needle decompression or insertion of a chest tube (according to protocol).

Abdominal Regions of the Body

Abdominal regions include the following:

      A = Right hypochondriac
      B = Epigastric (epi = on, above)
      C = Left hypochondriac
      D = Right lumbar
      E = Umbilical
      F = Left lumbar
      G = Right iliac
      H = Hypogastric (hypo = below, beneath, less than normal)
      I = Left iliac

The abdomen may also be divided into four quadrants (sections) with the umbilicus (navel) at the center: right upper quadrant (RUQ), right lower quadrant (RLQ), left upper quadrant (LUQ), and left lower quadrant (LLQ).

Peritoneal Spaces and the Anatomy of the Abdominal and Genitourinary Systems

The **peritoneum** lines the abdominal cavity. The anterior (front) area is the intraperitoneal space, which contains the stomach, the first part of the duodenum, the small intestines, and part of the large intestines and rectum as well as the liver, bile ducts, spleen, ovaries, part of the pancreas and ureters, and bladder. The posterior (back) retroperitoneal space contains part of the duodenum, the ascending and descending colon and part of the rectum as well as part of the pancreas and ureters, the kidneys, the adrenal glands, the uterus, and the fallopian tubes. The ovaries, uterus, and fallopian tubes comprise the female reproductive system. Solid organs include the liver, spleen, ovaries, uterus, pancreas, kidneys, and adrenals. Hollow organs include the bile ducts, stomach, large and small intestines, fallopian tubes, ureters, and bladder.

Abdominal Trauma

Abdominal trauma may result in blunt wounds, which may occur as the result of motor vehicle accidents, motorcycle accidents, pedestrian injuries, sports injuries, falls, blast injuries, and assaults. Blunt injuries comprise crush (compression), shear (tearing), and burst (sudden increased pressure) injuries. Motor vehicle accidents often result in liver injury in the passenger with impact on that side of the vehicle and spleen injury in the driver with impact on the driver's side. Other injuries from blunt trauma include damage to the diaphragm; retroperitoneal hematomas; and intestinal injuries, including perforation. Symptoms of internal injuries include pain, guarding, abdominal distension, discoloration, tenderness on movement, and evidence of lower rib fractures. Some may exhibit rectal bleeding and/or vomiting of blood. Prehospital: Provide airway/ventilation/oxygen supplementation as needed, place in a position of comfort, treat for shock if indicated (especially with suspected internal bleeding), and provide rapid transport for patients in an unstable condition.

Abdominal trauma may result in penetrating wounds, which are almost always related to gunshot wounds (high energy), shotgun wounds (medium energy), or knife wounds (low energy). Gunshot and shotgun wounds tend to cause more extensive damage than stab wounds, especially to the colon, liver, spleen, and diaphragm, and they may have an exit wound. Interior injuries may be extensive because the bullet damages tissues and may ricochet off of bone. Hemorrhage and peritonitis (especially with perforation of the intestines) are common complications. Pain is often more acute with injury to hollow organs than to solid organs, although blood loss may be severe with injury to the liver, spleen, or kidneys, and blood collecting in the retroperitoneal space may not be evident on inspection, palpation, or auscultation. Prehospital: Control external bleeding, manage the patient's airway/ventilation/oxygen supplementation, mobilize the spine if indicated, and apply a pneumatic antishock garment (PASG) if indicated for shock or pelvic fracture (contraindicated with difficulty breathing, pregnancy [second and third trimesters], evisceration, impaled object, and open fractures).

Eviscerations occur with open abdominal wounds, such as opening incisions or traumatic injuries, which allow the internal organs (often the intestines) to protrude externally. Surgical repair is required to reinsert the organs into the abdomen. The patient may go into shock, especially if the evisceration is part of other major injuries (common in trauma cases). Prehospital: Provide supportive care; cover the eviscerated organs with thick sterile gauze dressings moistened with NS, but do not attempt to reinsert the organs; manage the patient's airway/ventilation/oxygen supplementation as needed; and provide rapid transport. **Impalements** occur when an object penetrates the abdomen and remains in place and may be associated with multiple internal injuries and bleeding. Prehospital: Do not remove the object, but do expose the abdomen and manually secure the object with bulky dressings, and control any bleeding. Provide supportive care, manage the patient's airway/ventilation/oxygen supplementation as needed, and provide rapid transport.

Pneumatic Antishock Garment (PASG)

The **pneumatic antishock garment (PASG)** is indicated for hypovolemic shock and hypotension associated with and stabilization of pelvic and bilateral femur fractures. PASG is contraindicated with respiratory distress, pulmonary edema, pregnancy (second and third trimesters), heart failure, myocardial infarction, stroke, evisceration, abdominal or leg impalement, head injuries, and uncontrolled bleeding above the garment. PASG procedure is as follows:

- Place the garment flat on the patient-transport device/stretcher and transfer the patient onto the garment.
- If the patient is already on the stretcher, place the garment under his or her legs first and then lift the patient's buttocks and slide the garment upward until the upper garment edge is 1 inch below the bottom ribs.
- Secure the legs first and then the abdominal section with the Velcro straps.
- Attach the pump hoses to each leg and the abdominal section at the valves and close the stopcocks.
- Open the stopcock for each leg and abdominal section one at a time, and inflate them one at a time.
- After inflating each section, close the stopcock and check the vital signs. Stop inflating if the systolic BP ≥90 mm Hg. If the systolic BP is still < 90 mm Hg, then proceed to filling the next section until all three are filled.

Orthopedic Trauma

Fractures usually result from trauma (falls, auto accidents), but <u>pathologic fractures</u> can result from minor force to diseased bones (osteoporosis or cancerous lesions). <u>Stress fractures</u> are caused by repetitive trauma (forced marching). <u>Salter-Harris fractures</u> involve the cartilaginous epiphyseal plate near the ends of long bones in children who are growing, and this can impair bone growth. Fracture types are listed as follows:

- Open fractures with soft-tissue injury and a break in the skin overlying the fracture, including puncture wounds from external forces or bone fragments; these can result in osteomyelitis (bone infection).
- Closed fractures involve a broken bone but no break in the skin.

Symptoms include pain, deformity or angulation, swelling, bruising, inability to move the joint or bear weight, grating on movement, and impaired function or circulation. Isolated fractures are usually not life threatening, but pelvic and femur fractures may involve severe blood loss. Prehospital: Cover open wounds with sterile dressings, manually stabilize and immobilize the fracture area but do not replace protruding bones, apply a cold pack, place the patient in a position of comfort.

Subluxation (partial dislocation of a joint) and **luxation** (complete dislocation) can cause neurovascular compromise, which can be permanent if reduction is delayed. This is especially a problem with <u>hip dislocations</u>, which most commonly occur in automobile accidents when the person's knees impact the dashboard. <u>Elbow dislocations</u> often result from athletic injuries and may cause nerve damage. <u>Shoulder dislocations</u> are the most common type and also often result from athletic injuries. They may become chronic. <u>Knee dislocations</u> may result in severe injury to the popliteal artery, and this can lead to amputation, so rapid transport and emergent surgical repair are indicated. Differentiating between fractures and dislocations can be difficult because the symptoms and appearance are often similar. A deformity may not be evident, or it may be obscured by edema, or edema may give the appearance of a deformity. Extensive bruising may occur with all types of injuries, and pain may occur even with minor soft-tissue injuries. Prehospital: Splint and immobilize the area, apply a cold compress, and place the patient in a position of comfort.

Amputations may be partial or complete and result from crush, guillotine (cutting), or avulsion (twisting) injuries. A <u>simple amputation</u> requires no extrication and other injuries or shock are absent, but a <u>complex amputation</u> may involve multiple injuries, shock, and delayed treatment because of extrication. The amputated limb should be treated initially as though it could be reattached, although single digits (except the thumb) and lower limbs are not usually reattached. The part should be irrigated with normal saline (NS) to remove debris; wrapped in NS-moistened gauze; and placed in a sealed plastic bag, which should be immersed in ice water. The body part should not freeze and should not be placed directly on ice. Prehospital: Manage the patient's airway/ventilation/oxygen supplementation; control bleeding by using direct pressure or, if there is severe hemorrhage, by applying a BP cuff proximal to (above) the injury 70 mm Hg greater than the systolic BP for <30 minutes; irrigate the stump with NS if it is dirty; cover the open area with NS-moistened gauze; and elevate the stump.

Strains and Sprains

A **strain** is an overstretching of a part of the musculature ("pulled muscle") that causes microscopic tears in the muscle, usually resulting from excess stress or overuse of the muscle. The onset of pain is usually sudden with local tenderness on use of the muscle. A **sprain** is damage to a joint, with a partial rupture of the supporting ligaments and/or tendons, usually caused by wrenching or twisting that may occur with a fall. The rupture can damage blood vessels, resulting in edema, tenderness at the joint, and pain on movement with pain increasing over 2–3 hours after the injury. An avulsion fracture (the bone fragment is pulled away by a ligament) may occur with strain. Prehospital: Immobilize the area for transport, use rest, ice, compression, and elevation (the RICE protocol), and monitor the patient's neurovascular status (especially for sprains) by checking the pulse, capillary refill, color, and sensation distal to (below) the injury.

Pelvic Fractures

Pelvic fractures represent about 3% of total fractures, but they pose a greater risk than most other types of fractures. Pelvic fractures most often result from a motor vehicle accident (50%–60%) in adults and a pedestrian/motor vehicle impact (60%–80%) in children. Pelvic fractures may be accompanied by major injuries to soft tissue and internal organs, especially the bladder, urethra (especially in children and women), and colon. A fracture on one side often results in a fracture on the other side as well. The primary cause of death after a pelvic fracture is hemorrhage with between 50% and 70% of patients with unstable fractures requiring multiple transfusions. Geriatric patients have higher mortality rates than do younger patients. Symptoms include pain and tenderness, bloody urine, rectal bleeding, vaginal bleeding, hematoma over the fracture site, pain on hip motion, and signs of shock (with blood loss). Prehospital: Monitor vital signs for indications of shock, apply PASG or a pelvic wrap device (per protocol) to stabilize and prevent excessive movement, and monitor the patient's airway/ventilation/oxygen supplementation.

Types of Fractures

	Transverse: Usually occurs in long bones and is at risk of displacement unless it is splinted to prevent movement. Most often occurs from direct impact, such as sports injuries. May suggest abuse if occurring in small children.
	Comminuted: Usually results from high-impact trauma, such as with motor vehicle accidents, and it is more common in older adults or those with weakened bones. This fracture is very painful and is often accompanied by swelling and muscle spasms.
	Spiral: Common in toddlers who fall on an extended leg, breaking the tibia, but it may also occur with abuse in small children as a result of jerking on or twisting an extremity (usually the arm).
	Displaced: Poses a risk of damage to surrounding tissues, including nerves and blood vessels, and may lead to an open fracture if not properly splinted. Usually the deformity is evident.
	Greenstick: Most common in children whose bones are less hard. It is usually quite painful but without deformity.

Prehospital Management of Fractures

Fracture	Prehospital
Tibia/Fibula (lower leg)	Manually immobilize during splinting. Splint the joint above and below the fracture(s) (upper thigh to ankle) with a padded rigid long-leg splint or a pneumatic splint, and then secure it to the other leg for additional support.
Shoulder	Apply a sling to the affected side and secure the patient's arm against the body with a swathe to limit movement.
Knee	If the pulse below the fracture is adequate and there is no deformity, splint with the knee straight. If there is deformity, splint the leg in the position it was found. If there is no pulse below the fracture, consult with medical assistance immediately. Never use a traction splint.
Clavicle (upper chest)	Apply a sling to the affected side. (Common in young children who fall with an arm outstretched.)
Humerus (upper arm)	Apply a sling to the affected side and swathe the arm to the body to limit movement.
Radius/Ulna (forearm)	Splint from the elbow to the wrist and secure above and below the fracture. Elevate arm.
Elbow	Apply a sling to the affected side (often results from a fall).

Femur/Hip Fractures

The femur is the long bone in the thigh. Although any part of the femur may fracture, fractures in the upper femur are common and are generally referred to as hip fractures. **Femur fractures** in young patients usually result from high-impact trauma, such as motor vehicle or pedestrian/motor vehicle accidents, whereas femur fractures in geriatric patients are most often from falls and are associated with osteoporosis. Patients may have many comorbidities and may present with dehydration and blood loss. Mortality rates for hip fractures are high, with 10% during initial treatment and 25% over the next year. Symptoms of femur fractures include pain and deformity at

- 95 -

the fracture site and an inability to walk or bear weight. A hematoma may be present. Prehospital: Splint the leg in the position it was found in with a traction splint (Hare Traction Splint/Sager Emergency Traction Splint), flush open fractures with NS to remove debris, and apply an NS-moistened sterile gauze dressing, monitor vital signs and neurovascular status, and assess soft tissue for damage.

Assessment of Musculoskeletal Injuries and the Types of Splints

Assessment of musculoskeletal injuries should include the following:

- Palpation/Inspection for tissue damage, swelling, deformity, tenderness.
- Comparison with the opposite side if a limb is involved.
- Assessment of neurovascular status (pulse, color, sensation, function) distal to (below) the fracture.
- Assessment of the six P's: <u>pain</u> (site of pain, degree, character), <u>pallor</u> (below the fracture or generalized), <u>paresthesia</u> (impaired sensation below the fracture), distal <u>pulses</u> (intact, weak, absent), <u>paralysis</u> (with or without impaired sensation), and <u>pressure</u> (often associated with swelling and pain).
- Assessment of age and general condition (geriatric patients are more likely to have fractures from minor injuries because of osteoporosis).

If fracture or dislocation is suspected, then the area should be splinted or immobilized for transport. **Types of splints** include rigid (should be padded), nonrigid (moldable), traction, air (pneumatic devices), pillow/blanket, short spine board, and long spine board. Splinting procedures are similar for adults, pediatric patients, and geriatric patients.

Open Soft-Tissue Injuries

Injury	Characteristics	Prehospital
Abrasion	Painful superficial scraping of the outermost layer of skin. There is little or no bleeding.	Irrigate with water or NS to remove debris and cover with nonadherent dressing.
Laceration	A cut or break in the skin from impact with a sharp object. Bleeding may vary from mild to severe.	Apply pressure to control the bleeding, irrigate to remove debris if necessary, and cover with a dry sterile gauze dressing.
Puncture	Wound from impact with a sharp pointed object (knife, bullet); it may exhibit little external bleeding but major internal bleeding and soft-tissue damage. An exit wound may be present.	Apply pressure to control any bleeding, manage the patient's airway/ventilation/oxygen supplementation, and provide rapid transport if the patient's condition is unstable.
Impaled object	Penetrating object remains in wound.	Leave the object in place and pad with bulky dressings.
Foreign body in the eye(s)	Patient has pain; tearing; redness; and blurred or impaired vision from dirt, dust, chemicals or other materials in the eye(s).	Cover both eyes loosely (avoiding pressure) to prevent movement. If it is chemical contamination, flush the eye(s) with copious amounts of NS or water.

Closed Soft-Tissue Injuries

Injury	Characteristics	Prehospital
Contusion	Results from blunt or compressive pressure to a muscle and is a common sports injury. These may include other injuries, such as sprains, strains, fractures, and damage to internal organs. Symptoms include tenderness, pain on movement, and bruising. If bruising is in the shape of an instrument, it usually indicates abuse.	Provide RICE and supportive care.
Hematoma	Collection of blood within the tissue because of damaged blood vessels from injury, underlying fracture, or medications (such as warfarin). These may be small or very large, and patients may lose ≥1 of blood. Symptoms may include pain and swelling.	Provide supportive care for small contusions (which often resolve spontaneously), provide RICE therapy, and monitor for signs of continued bleeding.
Crush injury	External pressure may cause severe internal injuries, such as fractures and organ rupture.	Manage the patient's airway/ ventilation/oxygen supplementation and shock as needed, control bleeding, and provide supportive care.

Classification of Burns and the Rule of Nines

Burn injuries may be chemical, electrical, or thermal and are assessed by the area affected, percentage of the body burned, and the depth of the burn, as follows:

- First-degree burns are superficial and affect the epidermis, causing erythema and pain.
- Second-degree burns extend through the dermis (partial thickness), resulting in blistering and sloughing of the epidermis.
- Third-degree burns affect the underlying tissue, including the vasculature, muscles, and nerves (full thickness).

Burns are classified according to the American Burn Association's criteria as follows:

- Minor: <10% body surface area (BSA) or 2% BSA with third-degree burns without serious risk to the face, hands, feet, or perineum.
- Moderate: 10%–20% BSA combined second- and third-degree burns in adults; age <10 years or ≤10% third-degree without serious risk to the face, hands, feet, or perineum.
- Major: 20% BSA; ≥10% third-degree burns; all burns are to the face, hands, feet, or perineum and will result in functional/cosmetic defect; or burns with inhalation or other major trauma.

The rule of nines estimates the BSA burned: Adults—head 9%, trunk (front) 18%, trunk (back) 18%, arm 9%, leg 18%, perineum 1%. Infants/Children—head 18%, trunk (front) 18%, trunk (back) 18%, arm 9%, leg 13.5%, perineum 1%.

Management of Burns

Those with severe burns may develop shock and impairment of all major body systems. If the burning process is ongoing (smoldering clothes, tissue), room-temperature water or NS should be applied to stop the burning and any smoldering clothes or jewelry should be removed, although if the clothing is adhered to the skin, it should be left in place. Facial or airway burns are a major concern, so the airway must be monitored constantly with interventions as necessary. The burned area should be covered with nonadherent clean, dry dressings, and the patient should be kept warm for transport. Children experience greater fluid and heat loss because of their greater body surface area relative to their size, and the EMT should be alert to the possibility of child abuse. With **chemical burns**, any dry powder should be brushed off and wet chemicals should be flushed with copious amounts of water (by an EMT wearing gloves and eye protection). With **electrical burns**, internal burns may be more severe than external burns, and the patient is at risk of cardiac arrest.

Dressings and Bandages

Dressing/Bandage	Characteristics
Sterile gauze	4×4 (sponge) or roller/wrapping gauze (Kerlix) that is used to protect skin or pack wounds to control bleeding. Roller gauze may be used to secure other dressings.
Nonadherent dressings	Designed not to stick to open wounds because of their special coating (Teflon, foam, petrolatum, hydrogel). Used on abrasions, burns, and lightly draining wounds.
Occlusive dressings	These have a waxy coating to make an air- and water-tight seal, but they are not as absorbent as gauze. Used for sucking chest wounds, abdominal eviscerations, and lacerations of the external jugular vein or carotid.
Trauma dressings	Dressings that often include a nonadherent pad, clotting agent embedded in the dressing, and elastic wrap in one piece so that they can be rapidly applied (such as an ACE bandage); these include QuikClot Combat Gauze and Celox Rapid hemostatic gauze. Especially useful to control bleeding and to apply pressure to a wound.
Adhesive, roller bandages	May be elastic or nonelastic, and they are used to secure other dressings and/or apply compression.

Head Injuries

Injury	Characteristics	Prehospital
Head	Open: Bleeding. Closed: Swelling and bruising, may have depression of the skull and underlying injury. Battle's sign (bruising over the mastoid process) and/or raccoon eyes (bruising about the eyes) may indicate a basal skull fracture.	Apply direct pressure to control the bleeding; apply dry, sterile dressings. Monitor the patient's mental status. Be alert for signs of skull fracture.
Scalp	Copious bleeding may occur. May cause shock in infants and young children. Injuries above the ears increase the risk of brain injury.	As above. Manage the patient's airway/ventilation/oxygen supplementation if needed. Rapid transport is required with shock. Avoid closing the patient's mouth with bandages.
Facial	May include soft-tissue damage, facial bone fractures (nasal, orbital), eye injuries, and oral/dental injuries (tooth avulsions, mandibular/maxillary fractures). May have severe swelling, airway compromise, impaired vision, and bloody nose.	Maintain a patent airway, but avoid nasopharyngeal airways; suction as needed; take broken teeth to the hospital; examine the eyes; and control bleeding. Patch both eyes if one or both eyes are injured. Stabilize impaled objects in the eye(s), but remove impaled objects from the cheeks if any bleeding obstructs the patient's airway.

Brain and Cervical Spine Injuries

Injury	Characteristics	Prehospital
Brain	Direct injury to brain tissue or damage from bleeding inside of the skull may occur, resulting in altered mental status. Cerebrospinal fluid may leak from the nose/ears. Symptoms include the pupils being unequal, nausea and/or vomiting, bradycardia (slow heart rate), increased BP, and irregular breathing. Contusions (bruising) may cause microhemorrhages.	Immobilize the spine; manage the patient's airway/ventilation/oxygen supplementation; provide shock prevention; control bleeding; provide rapid transport.
Spine	Suspect with motor vehicle/pedestrian accidents; falls; hanging; blunt or penetrating trauma to head, neck or torso; diving accidents, and unresponsive trauma patients. May have tenderness in the area; pain on moving; numbness, tingling, or weakness; the inability to feel or move below the injury; difficulty breathing; and incontinence (bowel and/or bladder).	Responsive: Manually stabilize the head and neck in the position found until a cervical collar and backboard are in place. Question the patient's pain, sensations, and ability to move. Unresponsive: Stabilize the head and neck as above; manage the airway, ventilation, and oxygenation; question witnesses; and provide rapid transport.

Anatomy of the Brain and Spinal Cord

The **brain** is protected by the skull and the meninges, and three layers of lining: the dura mater, arachnoid mater, and the pia mater. Brain tissue is comprised of gray matter (neurons [nerve cells]) and white matter (covered nerve pathways that conduct messages). The main part of the brain is the cerebrum, which is comprised of two hemispheres that contain the frontal parietal, temporal, and occipital lobes. The cerebrum controls higher brain functions, including thoughts, speech, vision, hearing, and actions. The cerebellum lies in the back of the brain below the cerebellum and controls equilibrium and coordination. The brain stem controls involuntary functions, such as respirations, heart rate, temperature control, and nerve transmission. The brain stem is continuous with the **spinal cord**, which is also protected by the meninges and the vertebrae (cervical, thoracic, and lumbar). Cerebrospinal fluid circulates within the subarachnoid space of the brain and the spinal cord.

Intracranial Hematomas

Type	Characteristics	Prehospital
Epidural	Bleeding between the dura and the skull, pushing the brain downward and inward. The hemorrhage is usually caused by arterial tears, so bleeding is often rapid, leading to severe neurological deficits and respiratory arrest. Patient may be lucid and without symptoms for 2–6 hours after the injury.	Provide supportive care, keep the patient's head elevated to reduce intracranial pressure, note neurological status (movement, strength, mental status, pupils equal and reactive or unequal/fixed), and provide rapid transport.
Subdural	Bleeding between the dura and the arachnoid mater, usually from tears in the cortical veins of the subdural space. It tends to develop more slowly than an epidural hemorrhage. If the bleeding is acute and develops within minutes or hours of injury, then the prognosis is poor. Subacute hematomas that develop more slowly cause varying degrees of injury.	
Intracerebral	Bleeding into the substance of the brain from an artery. Sudden onset; it results in a hemorrhagic stroke with a lack of nutrients and oxygen to parts of the brain. May result from degenerative changes, hypertension, brain tumors, medications, or illicit drugs (crack, cocaine). Symptoms vary depending on the site, but they may include one-sided weakness, paralysis, difficult speaking, severe headache, and altered mental status.	Provide supportive care, keep the patient's head elevated to reduce intracranial pressure, note neurological status (movement, strength, mental status, pupils equal and reactive or unequal/fixed), and provide rapid transport

Subarachnoid	Bleeding in the space between the meninges and brain and into the cerebrospinal fluid, usually resulting from an aneurysm, arteriovenous malformation (AVM), or trauma. This type of hemorrhage compresses the brain tissue. The first presenting symptoms are severe headache, nausea and vomiting, nuchal rigidity, palsy related to cranial nerve compression, retinal hemorrhages, and papilledema.	

Concussion

Concussion is a brain injury in which structural damage is not apparent but neurological functioning is impaired. Patients may experience a brief loss of consciousness after a head injury and may experience confusion and even bizarre behavior (if the frontal lobe is affected). Other symptoms include severe headache, somnolence, dizziness, lack of coordination, confusion, disorientation, inappropriate emotional response, nausea, and vomiting. Symptoms are usually transient (lasting from minutes to hours), but up to 50% may have recurrent symptoms (such as difficulty concentrating, headaches, and dizziness) for months.

The American Academy of Neurology classifies concussions as follows:

- Grade 1: Transient confusion without loss of consciousness with symptoms resolving in <15 minutes.
- Grade 2: Transient confusion without loss of consciousness with symptoms resolving in >15 minutes.
- Grade 3: Any loss of consciousness of any duration.

Prehospital: Provide supportive care and reassurance, monitor vital signs and neurological status for signs of increasing intracranial pressure that may indicate more severe injury, and elevate the patient's head.

Signs of Increasing Intracranial Pressure

Head trauma may result in **increased intracranial pressure** and cerebral edema. Patients often suffer initial hypertension, which increases intracranial pressure and decreases perfusion, and significant swelling, which also interferes with perfusion, causing hypoxia and hypercapnia (increased carbon dioxide), which trigger increased blood flow. This increased volume at a time when injury impairs autoregulation further increases cerebral edema, which, in turn, increases intracranial pressure and results in a further decrease in perfusion with resultant ischemia (impaired circulation). If the pressure continues to rise, the brain may herniate. Symptoms include Cushing's triad: wide pulse pressure, bradycardia, and irregular respirations. Initially: Decreased levels of consciousness, increased BP, and decreased pulse, Cheyne-Stokes (irregular) respirations, pupils reactive. Middle brain stem involvement: Wide pulse pressure, bradycardia, pupils sluggish or nonreactive, hyperventilation. Lower brain stem: Pupil blown on the side of injury, irregular respirations, flaccid response to painful stimulation, and BP and pulse decrease. Prehospital: Elevate the patient's head, manage the patient's airway/ventilation/oxygen supplementation, and provide rapid transport.

Nonspinal Neck Injuries and Nasal Fractures

Nonspinal neck injuries may result from blunt trauma or penetrating trauma, and they must be carefully assessed for underlying spinal cord injury. Open wounds may bleed profusely, especially if the carotid artery is breached, resulting in rapid exsanguination and death. The airway may be compromised. Difficulty swallowing indicates esophageal injury, whereas voice changes indicate laryngeal injury. Crackling on palpation indicates air in the tissues. Prehospital: Apply single-digit (gloved) pressure to control bleeding of the carotid artery or jugular veins; apply an occlusive dressing for an injury to large vessels after the bleeding is controlled to prevent air from entering the bloodstream, which is life-threatening; and manage the patient's airway/ventilation/oxygen supplementation (advanced life support may be needed). Rapid or air medical transport may be needed. **Nasal fractures** (40% of facial fractures) may cause persistent bleeding and should be assessed for drainage of the cerebrospinal fluid and injury of the surrounding structures, including brain injury, skull fracture, and neck and cervical spine injury. Prehospital: Control any bleeding, elevate the patient's head, and manage the airway but do not use nasopharyngeal airways.

Facial and Dental Injuries

Facial injuries may include soft-tissue injuries, fractures, and eye injuries. Facial fractures may result in airway obstruction, pain, swelling, bruising, deformation, and bleeding. Fractures of the maxilla and mandible (the upper and lower jaw) often result in damage to the teeth as well. **Dental fractures,** most commonly of the maxillary teeth, may occur in association with other oral and facial injuries and may be overlooked unless a careful dental examination is carried out. Fractures may range from chipping of the enamel to fracture of the tooth root. **Dental avulsions** are complete displacement of a tooth from its socket. The tooth may be reimplanted if done within 1–2 hours after displacement, although only permanent teeth are reimplanted, not primary teeth, so question the parents of children to determine if an avulsed tooth is permanent. Prehospital: Manage the patient's airway/ventilation/oxygen supplementation as needed, elevate the patient's head, and place the avulsed tooth in NS for transport.

Mandibular Fractures, Laryngotracheal Injuries, and Non-CNS-Associated Spinal Trauma

Mandibular fractures are most common in males 21 to 30 and result from a blow to the jaw from an assault, motor vehicle accident, or gunshot wound and are often associated with other injuries, such as head injury or midface fractures. Symptoms include malocclusion of teeth, pain, point tenderness, and ecchymosis of the floor of the mouth. Prehospital: Manage the patient's airway/ventilation/oxygen supplementation (avoid the nasal airway), use an ice pack to reduce edema, elevate the patient's head, and monitor him or her closely.

Laryngotracheal injuries result from direct trauma and may result in swelling and hemorrhage. Symptoms include swelling, changes in voice, hemoptysis, subcutaneous emphysema (from open wounds), and structural irregularities. The patient must be assessed for associated injuries. Prehospital: Manage the patient's airway/ventilation/oxygen supplementation because airway obstruction is common, elevate the patient's head, and provide supportive care. The patient may require a surgical airway.

With **non-CNS-associated spinal trauma,** patients complain of pain and point tenderness, but neurological findings are intact. Prehospital: Provide sitting or standing spinal mobilization and supportive care; manage the patient's airway/ventilation/oxygen supplementation as needed.

Anatomy and Physiology of the Eye and Eye Conditions

The **eyes** fit into sockets (orbits) in the skull. The eyelid and sclera are lined with conjunctiva (clear tissue). The outer layer of the eye is the cornea, which focuses light. The pupil (at the center) dilates or constricts to control light coming into the eye. The iris (the colored part) adjusts the size of the pupil. The lens is behind the pupil and allows the eyes to focus. The vitreous humor is the gel-like substance in the middle of the globe. The retina at the back of the eye transmits visual images to the brain. The sclera (white part) contains blood vessels and protects the eye.

Eye conditions		
Condition	**Characteristics**	**Prehospital**
Burns	Chemical/fire: Pain, tearing, difficulty opening the affected eye.	Irrigate with NS or sterile water for 20–30 minutes.
Corneal abrasion (scratch)/ Foreign body	Often associated with a failure to use safety glasses or wearing contact lenses. A foreign body may remain in the eye(s). Symptoms: Blurred vision, pain, tearing, photophobia, and squinting (muscle spasms).	As above. Do not attempt to remove a foreign body; patch both eyes to prevent movement.

Orbital Fractures and Perforated Tympanic Membrane

Orbital fractures most often occur with blunt force against the globe causing a rupture through the floor of the orbital bone or a direct blow to the orbital rim, often related to an assault or sports injury. Injuries are most common in adolescents and young adults. Patients may be essentially asymptomatic, or they may exhibit ecchymosis and edema of the eyelid, infraorbital anesthesia from pressure or damage to the infraorbital nerve, decreased sensation of the cheek and upper gum on the injured side, diplopia (double vision), and enophthalmos (sunken globe). Prehospital: Patch both eyes to prevent movement, provide supportive care, and use an ice compress to reduce edema.

A **ruptured tympanic membrane** may result from pressure (diving, waterskiing), a direct blow to the ear, explosions, and a foreign object in the ear. Symptoms may include pain, hemorrhagic otorrhea (bloody drainage), and hearing impairment. Prehospital: Provide supportive care.

Skull Fractures

The skull is divided into eight cranial bones: one frontal bone (over the frontal lobe), two parietal bones (over the parietal lobes), two temporal bones (over the temporal lobes), one occipital bone (over the occipital lobe and cerebellum), one sphenoid bone (it forms part of the eye orbit), and one ethmoid bone (it separates the nasal cavity from the brain). **Skull fractures** include the following:

- Basilar: Occurs in the bones at the base of the brain and can cause severe brain stem damage.
- Comminuted: The skull fractures into small pieces.
- Compound: A surface laceration extends to a skull fracture, which may be overlooked because of heavy bleeding.
- Depressed: May be open and is often comminuted. Pieces of the skull are depressed inward on the brain tissue, often producing dural tears and underlying brain trauma.
- Linear/hairline: A skull fracture forms a thin line without any splintering, usually without any underlying injury.
- Diastatic: Affects children younger than 3 years old, widening the skull sutures.

Spinal Injuries and Spinal Cord Injuries

Spinal injuries of the vertebrae include fractures, dislocations, open wounds, and flexion and extension injuries. Because the spinal cord lies within the vertebral column, injury to the vertebrae may cause **spinal cord injuries** and disrupt transmissions in nerves that connect the body and the brain. Spinal cord injuries may affect only a few nerves, or they may completely transect the spinal cord, resulting in permanent paralysis below the site of injury. Spinal cord injuries should be suspected with head trauma, penetrating trauma, direct blunt trauma, falls, diving injuries, motor vehicle accidents, rapid deceleration accidents, and multisystem trauma. Assessment includes evaluating extremity movement, respiration control, sensation, pain/tenderness, and vital signs. Prehospital: Logroll the patient to examine his or her back, immobilize the patient (seated or standing), apply a rigid cervical collar, lift and move him or her with care, and provide rapid transport. Elevate the torso of children 2–3 cm with padding so that the head is in a neutral position if using an adult immobilization device. Immobilize infants in their car seats, padding all the voids.

Brain Injuries, the Coup/Contrecoup Pattern, and Posturing

Primary brain injuries are those that result from the original trauma and include direct damage to brain tissue, such as may occur with a gunshot wound. **Secondary brain injuries** result from the effects of the primary injury, such as increasing intracranial pressure, ischemia (most common), hemorrhage, edema, and brain herniation. **Coup/Contrecoup** injuries are common in motor vehicle accidents and shaken baby syndrome. With acceleration/deceleration and contact injuries where the head hits a fixed object (such as a windshield) and snaps back from the impact, *coup* (on the side of impact) and contrecoup (on the opposite side) contusions may both occur. **Decerebrate (extension) posturing** (with the body stiff, legs straight, feet extended, arms straight, and the head/neck arched back) is associated with severe midbrain damage. **Decorticate (flexion) posturing** (with the body stiff, legs straight, and hands clenched on the chest) is associated with damage to the pathway connecting the brain and spinal cord and may include damage to the cerebral cortex, white matter, or basal ganglia.

Pregnancy Trauma

The mother and fetus are each considered to be patients. Trauma is the cause of 46% of maternal deaths, and blunt trauma is the cause of up to 38% of fetal deaths. Pregnant patients are susceptible to falls (especially in the third trimester when the mother's center of gravity shifts) and domestic abuse (which may include blunt trauma and penetrating trauma from knife or gunshot wounds). However, most trauma in pregnant women occurs as the result of motor vehicle accidents. Pregnant women have an increased blood volume and heart rate, impaired venous return if in a supine (flat) position in the third trimester, and increased risk of vomiting and aspiration. Hypovolemia/shock reduces the amount of oxygen to the fetus, resulting in fetal stress. Vaginal bleeding may occur. Prehospital: Have suction available, monitor the patient's airway/ventilation/oxygen supplementation, and provide 100% oxygen per nonrebreather mask and ventilation assistance if needed (especially with symptoms of shock), transport on the left side (tilt the immobilization board if necessary), and provide rapid transport.

Pediatric Trauma

Note the pediatric assessment triangle (appearance, work of breathing, and circulation). Respiration rates vary with age, but the use of accessory muscles and sternal retraction indicate respiratory distress. Assess the brachial pulse in infants—a slow pulse indicates hypoxia. Trauma is the leading cause of death in pediatric patients, and hypoventilation is the leading cause of cardiac arrest. BP values are not reliable for small children, who may have normal BP in compensated shock. <u>Shaken baby syndrome</u> should be considered with pediatric trauma; it is believed to be the result of vigorous shaking of an infant, causing acute subdural hematoma (brain hemorrhage) and retinal (eye) hemorrhages. It is believed that the shaking of the brain causes coup (front) and contrecoup (back) damage as well as damaging the vessels and nerves with resultant cerebral edema (swelling). Prehospital: Manage hypovolemia/shock, prevent hypothermia, and manage the patient's airway/ventilation/oxygen supplementation as needed. Ventilate if the patient is bradycardic. BVM ventilation is usually the best ventilation method for children.

Geriatric Trauma

These patients are more susceptible to trauma because of aging processes, and they may be less able to maintain normal vital signs during hemorrhage. About 80% of patients older than age 65 have one chronic illness, and 50% have two. Polypharmacy is common, and medications may affect vital signs and blood clotting. Response times may be slower than normal Falls are the most common cause of injury in geriatric patients. Elder abuse should be suspected if patients have repeated injuries. Scalding is the most common burn injury and is often deeper because of thinning skin. The risk of cerebral bleeding with trauma is increased because of brain shrinkage. The cough reflex may be lessened. Fractures are common because of osteoporosis, especially hip fractures. Prehospital: Splint fractures, monitor the patient's airway/ventilation/oxygen supplementation, monitor oxygenation with pulse oximetry, suction if necessary, and check the mouth for dentures (which may obstruct the airway). Note: Spinal curvature may require padding of the spinal board.

Trauma in Cognitively Impaired Patients

Disorders may include Alzheimer's or other forms of dementia, traumatic brain injuries, strokes, Down's syndrome, and autistic spectrum disorders, so patients may be of all ages. Patients may be more at risk of trauma, and assessment and history taking may be difficult. Perceptions of pain may be altered, and psychological reactions may vary. Patients who are cognitively impaired are often more vulnerable to physical, sexual, and psychological abuse and may be unable to or afraid to report abuse. Patients may have an exaggerated response to pain or injury and may be very frightened and agitated or withdrawn, so the extent of the injury may be difficult to determine. Prehospital: Remain supportive, reassure the patient, avoid any use of medical jargon, use simple statements (asking one question at a time), use yes/no questions, obtain information from the caregiver if necessary, and treat as indicated by the patient's condition.

Generalized Hypothermia

Generalized hypothermia occurs when the body temperature falls to below-normal levels.

- Mild: 32°C–35°C (89.6°F–95°F).
- Moderate: 28°C–32°C (82.4 °F–95°F).
- Severe: <32°C (<82.4°F).

Contributing factors include wet and cold environments, wind, age (geriatric/pediatric), medical conditions, substance abuse (alcohol, drugs), and poison. Up to 50% of trauma patients with severe injuries become hypothermic because of exposure, blood loss, shock, and standard procedures (such as administration of cold fluids and clothing removal). Indications of hypothermia include cold skin, shivering, decreased mental status (confusion, memory loss, lethargy, dizziness, mood changes, impaired judgment, difficulty speaking), decreased sensation of touch, decreased motor function (muscle rigidity, stiff posture, muscle/joint stiffness), and bradycardia (slow pulse).

Prehospital: Remove the patient from the cold environment, remove any wet clothing, wrap in warm blankets, begin CPR if no pulse is obtained after 30–45 seconds of assessment, and use an AED if it indicates the need to defibrillate.

Decompression Sickness

Decompression sickness (dysbarism) occurs when a diver ascends too quickly and the body is unable to compensate for the pressure change. Because the pressure reduces too rapidly, dissolved gases in the blood, such as helium and nitrogen, form bubbles. These bubbles interfere with blood flow and can cause gas emboli, which can obstruct blood vessels and damage the alveoli in the lung. The gas emboli can affect all tissues, with symptoms ranging from mild to severe to complete neurological and cardiovascular collapse. Typical mild to moderate symptoms include joint pain, numbness, tremors, amnesia, difficulty breathing, itch, tinnitus, vertigo, and localized swelling. Severe symptoms include pneumothorax, loss of consciousness, seizures, weakness, or paralysis of extremities. Onset of mild symptoms is gradual with more than 40% having symptoms within one hour, but the onset of severe symptoms may occur within minutes of surfacing. Prehospital: Rapid transport for recompression therapy is critical to survival (especially in severe cases); manage the patient's airway/ventilation/oxygen supplementation with 100% oxygen through a nonrebreather mask. Air transport must be below 1000 feet in altitude.

Heat-Related Illnesses

Condition	Characteristics	Prehospital
Heat stress	Increased temperature causes dehydration. Symptoms may include swelling of the hands and feet, flushing, itching, sunburn, dizziness, muscle cramps, and hyperventilation. The patient's temperature is normal.	Remove the patient from heat, give fluids to rehydrate, and give oxygen with a nonrebreather mask.
Heat exhaustion	Dehydration results in sodium depletion. Symptoms may include flu-like symptoms, headache, dizziness, fainting, nausea, vomiting, weakness, muscle cramping, rapid pulse, diaphoresis, and cold clammy skin. The patient's temperature is usually <106°F (41°C), and it may be normal.	Remove the patient from heat; use evaporative cooling techniques such as ice packs to the axilla, groin, and neck; and rehydrate (one-half glass of fluid every 15 to 20 minutes). Give oxygen as above.
Heat stroke	There are two types, which may progress to multiorgan dysfunction syndrome with liver and kidney failure, and death. <u>Exertional:</u> Sudden onset after exertion. The patient's temperature varies because he or she is still sweating; there is diaphoresis, syncope, and loss of consciousness. <u>Nonexertional:</u> Sudden onset after heat exposure. The temperature is usually >106°F (41°C) rectally or >103°F (39.4°C) orally. There can be mild irritability, decorticate posturing, seizures, coma, and tachycardia.	Remove the patient from heat, apply evaporative cooling and ice packs as above, provide airway/ventilation/oxygenation support as needed, and provide rapid transport.

Frostbite/Freezing

Frostbite is tissue damage from **freezing**, most often affecting the nose, ears, and distal extremities (hands/feet). The affected part feels numb and aches or throbs, becoming hard and insensate as the tissue freezes, resulting in circulatory impairment, necrosis of tissue, and gangrene. Degrees of frostbite/freezing are as follows:

1. Partial freezing with redness and mild swelling, stinging, burning, and throbbing pain.
2. Full-thickness freezing with increased swelling in 3–4 hours and clear blisters in 6–24 hours; sloughing of skin with eschar formation, numbness, and then aching and throbbing pain.
3. Full-thickness freezing into the subdermal tissue with cyanosis, hemorrhagic blisters, skin necrosis, a "wooden" feeling, severe burning, throbbing, and shooting pains.
4. Freezing extends into the subcutaneous tissue (muscles, tendons, and bones) with a mottled appearance, nonblanching cyanosis, and eventually deep black eschar.

Prehospital: Remove the patient from the cold environment, handling him or her with care; remove wet clothing; cover the patient with a blanket; remove jewelry; manually stabilize the affected area; and transport rapidly. Do NOT break blisters, rub or massage the area, apply heat, rewarm if the area may refreeze, allow the patient to walk, or give him or her anything by mouth.

Submersion/Drowning

Submersion may cause aspiration (wet drowning) or trigger severe laryngospasm (dry drowning), although some people will be pulled from the water still breathing. **Drowning** is the leading cause of death in children younger than age 5, and it is the second leading cause of death in children younger than age 15. Most infant submersions are in bathtubs and result from intentional injury or lack of supervision. Adolescent/Adult submersions are often related to drugs, alcohol, or risk-taking behaviors. Submersion asphyxiation can cause profound damage to multiple organ systems, including the brain, heart, and lungs, from lack of oxygen and aspiration. Hypothermia related to near drowning has some protective effect because blood is shunted to the brain and heart. Indications of submersion include coughing, vomiting, difficulty breathing, and respiratory and cardiac arrest. Prehospital: Initiate CPR if the patient is in arrest, manage the patient's airway/ventilation/oxygen supplementation with 100% oxygen (the patient may need intubation), place the patient in the recovery position if he or she is unconscious or vomiting, provide suction as needed, and provide rapid transport.

Insect Bites

Injury	Characteristics	Prehospital
Fire ants	Hives and blistering with severe itching, redness, pain, and burning. Some patients may develop systemic reactions and anaphylaxis.	Provide supportive care and cold compresses. Use the anaphylaxis protocol if necessary.
Wasps/ bees	Pain, itching, redness, and swelling (most common). Severe allergic (hives) and/or anaphylactic (life-threatening) reactions.	Wipe the area with gauze or scrape it with a sharp instrument to remove the stinger, wash with soap and water, apply ice, and elevate. Use the anaphylaxis protocol if necessary.

Scorpions	May cause local (burning, itching, pain, and redness) or severe neurologic and/or other systemic reaction, such as paresthesia, stroke, hypertension, tachycardia, respiratory distress, priapism, hemorrhage, nausea, and vomiting. Pregnant women may miscarry.	Immobilize the affected part below the level of the heart, apply cool compresses (the first 2 hours), monitor the patient's airway/ventilation/oxygen supplementation, and provide rapid transport.
Ticks	Pain may occur at the bite site. Ticks may carry numerous infections, including Lyme disease, so follow-up is essential.	Grasp the tick near the skin with tweezers and pull with steady upward pressure, disinfect the site, and save the tick in a plastic bag.

Spider Bites

Injury	Characteristics	Prehospital
Black widow	Initially there are two faint fang marks with a pale area surrounded by a red-blue ring. Muscle cramps, pain radiating to the upper chest (arm bites) or abdomen (leg bites) and weakness within 2 hours increasing to generalized pain, headache, itching chills, nausea, vomiting, dyspnea, hypertension, cardiac abnormalities, shock, and coma.	Provide supportive care and analgesia. Take the spider in a sealed plastic bag to the receiving facility.
Brown recluse	Red, swollen bite site with severe pain and itching; "red, white, and blue" sign—a pale center with a central blister and reddish-blue peripheral discoloration with the blister becoming ischemic and necrotic—leaving an open ulcerated area that covers with black eschar and may expand in size. The following systemic reactions may occur within 6–12 hours in some patients: fever, vomiting, jaundice, hypotension, change in mental status, hemolytic anemia, disseminated intravascular coagulation, renal failure, seizures, coma, and death.	

Snakebites

Pit vipers include rattlesnakes, copperheads, and cottonmouths. They have erectile fangs that fold until they are aroused; their venom is primarily hemotoxic and cytotoxic, but it may also have neurotoxic properties (affecting the blood, cells, and nerves at the bite site and systemically). Symptoms vary depending on the amount of venom that is injected (many bites are dry).

- Wounds usually show one or two fang marks.
- Swelling may begin immediately, or it may be delayed for up to 6 hours.
- Pain may be severe.
- There may be a wide range of symptoms, including hypotension and impairment of blood clotting that can lead to excessive blood loss, depending upon the type and amount of venom.
- Progressive weakness, vision problems, nausea and vomiting, altered consciousness, and seizures are expected.

- 108 -

Prehospital: Note the time elapsed from the time of the bite to the time of transport, reassure the patient, immobilize the extremity, cleanse the wound with soap and water, apply an ice pack to slow venous return and reduce swelling, transport immediately for further treatment such as with antivenom, and mark the extent of swelling on the skin every 15 minutes.

Electrical Injuries

Low-voltage **electrical contact** most often causes a localized burn (first to third degree) to the hand or mouth (toddlers) with various degrees of tissue damage, although mouth contact may also result in cardiac or respiratory arrest. High-voltage electrical contact results in an entry and an exit wound with internal damage occurring between these wounds. Electrical current takes the shortest route to leave the body (flowing along blood vessels and nerves), so if the current passes from hand to hand, damage is usually more severe than if it passes from a hand to a foot. Severe injury may result in damage to bones, compartment syndrome, organ failure, and cardiac arrest from asystole or ventricular fibrillation. Vessels may be mildly or severely damaged. Abdominal organs may be damaged. Neurological damage with unconsciousness is common, especially if the current passes through the head. Peripheral nerve damage is also common, and damage to the spinal cord may occur. Prehospital: Manage the patient's airway/ventilation/oxygen supplementation, provide CPR/defibrillation as needed, and provide rapid transport (with the head elevated if it was involved).

Lightning Injuries

Lightning injuries may occur with a direct strike (≤5%), side splash from a strike nearby, contact voltage when touching an item that has been struck, ground current (from a more distant strike), and blunt trauma from being too close to a strike (which often results in the patient being thrown). Symptoms may vary, but they can include external burns (Lichtenberg figures) in a fernlike pattern, acute pain, fixed and dilated pupils (temporary), eye injuries, confusion, headache, hearing loss, perforated eardrum, hypotension, paralysis/paresis, spinal cord injury, altered mental status, brain injury, fractures, and cardiac arrest. Patients may be responsive initially but lapse into unconsciousness as cerebral edema increases, resulting in secondary respiratory and/or cardiac arrest. Burns are usually mild because of the brief contact. Prehospital: Manage the patient's airway/ventilation/oxygen supplementation, provide CPR/defibrillation as needed, and provide rapid transport (with the head elevated).

Multisystem Trauma

Multisystem trauma (common) involves injury to more than one major system. Care includes the following points:

- Ensure the safety of the patient and all rescue personnel, and determine the need for additional resources.
- Consider the mechanism of injury and identify and manage life-threatening conditions.
- Manage the patient's airway/ventilation/oxygen supplementation (high concentration) as well as the necessary spinal immobilization with him or her in a lying/sitting position, and make positioning decisions.
- Control hemorrhage and provide shock therapy and maintain body temperature.
- Splint musculoskeletal injuries.
- Suspect additional injuries.
- Prioritize interventions and continue care en route rather than delaying transport.

- Evaluate the patient's condition by the injuries sustained (bleeding, difficulty breathing, lack of pulse) rather than by the patient's response (screaming, yelling).
- Complete the primary and secondary assessments, and obtain a medical history.
- Platinum ten—the first 10 minutes on the scene in which the patient should be extricated and stabilization efforts should be started.
- Golden hour—the first 60 minutes during which the patient should be stabilized and transported to the receiving facility.
- Notify the receiving facility so resources are prepared.

Blast Injuries

Blast injuries may result from high-order explosives (TNT, nitroglycerin) or low-order explosives (pipe bombs, Molotov cocktails). Enclosed explosions usually cause more injury than do open-air blasts. Blast waves occur only with high-order explosives and result from high-pressure impulses. Blast wind may occur with either type of explosives and involves superheated air. Ground shock may cause further injury. Immediate death may occur. Injuries may include the following:

Type	Characteristics	Prehospital
Primary	Blast wave injury affects gas-filled organs/structures: lungs, eardrum, abdomen, eyes, and brain (20% of victims).	Be alert for a second explosive device or a device on a victim (who may be a perpetrator).
Secondary	Penetrating injuries from flying shrapnel affecting any part of the body along with abrasions, contusions, and lacerations. (Secondary injury is the most common cause of death.)	Carry out rapid triage. Control any bleeding/manage shock. Manage the patient's airway/ventilation/
Tertiary	Injuries from being thrown by blast wind: fractures, spinal and brain injuries, and traumatic amputations.	oxygen supplementation. Provide CPR if necessary. Splint musculoskeletal
Quaternary	Other injuries and complications, such as difficulty breathing because of smoke inhalation, burns, and crush injuries.	injuries. Provide rapid transport.

Special Patient Populations

Premonitory Signs of Labor

Lightening	As the fetal head engages and moves toward the birth canal, the fundal pressure on the diaphragm lessens, so the mother can breathe more easily, but pressure in the pelvic area increases, causing urinary frequency. The lower abdomen may protrude more than previously. Increased circulatory impairment may cause venous stasis and ankle swelling as well as increased vaginal secretions as the vaginal mucous membranes become congested. Pressure on the nerves may result in leg cramps or pelvic and leg pain.
Braxton Hicks (BH)	BH contractions are short in duration, occur at irregular intervals in the lower abdomen, and do not change the cervix. They are often relieved by activity or mild analgesia. The intensity and frequency of BH contractions often increase immediately prior to the onset of true labor.
Cervical changes	The cervix ripens (softens) to allow for effacement (thinning) and dilation.
Bloody show	A mucous plug from pooled secretions forms at the opening of the cervical canal during pregnancy, and when the cervix begins to efface, this mucous plug is expelled, exposing capillary vessels that bleed. The bloody show typically appears as pink mucus. Bloody show usually occurs within 24 to 48 hours of the onset of labor.
Ruptured membranes	Rupture of the membranes occurs in about 12% of women prior to the onset of labor, which usually then occurs within 24 hours. Before rupture, the membranes typically bulge through the dilating cervix; fluid comes in a gush, although it may come in smaller spurts in some cases. If the membranes rupture before engagement of the fetal head, the umbilical cord may prolapse with the fluid, increasing risk to the fetus, so mothers should always seek medical attention after rupture. If the mother is at term and labor does not start within 24 hours of rupture, labor may be induced.

Stages of Labor

First	Latent phase: The cervix begins to dilate; contractions are mild to moderate and occur every 3–30 minutes and are of short duration. Active phase: The cervix is dilated to 4–7 cm; contractions are every 1–5 minutes, lasting 20–40 seconds. Pain is increased. Transitional phase: The cervix is fully dilated (8–10 cm); contractions come every 1.5–2 minutes, lasting 60–90 seconds. There is increased pain, hyperventilation, crying, moaning, vomiting, and rectal pressure.
Second	From fully dilated cervix to delivery with contractions as in the transitional phase. The perineum begins to bulge, and the fetal head crowns as the mother begins to bear down and birth is imminent. Pressure on the rectum and anus may cause stool to be expelled. Birth occurs head first if it is a normal delivery, feet first if it is a breech delivery.
Third	Delivery of the placenta should occur 5–30 minutes after birth. Retained placenta occurs if more than 30 minutes elapse.
Fourth	The period of 1–4 hours after birth, which involves 250–400 mL blood loss, moderate hypotension (low BP), and tachycardia (rapid pulse).

- 111 -

Organs of Pregnancy and Vaginal Bleeding

Organs of pregnancy include the uterus (womb). The placenta is attached to the walls of the uterus; it includes the umbilical cord, which provides blood, nutrients, and oxygen to the fetus. The fetus is inside an amniotic sac, which contains amniotic fluid that cushions the fetus. The opening to the uterus is the cervix, which thins and dilates for delivery. The vagina provides the birth canal.

Vaginal bleeding during the first trimester of pregnancy may indicate spontaneous abortion, ectopic pregnancy, or infection, although light occasional spotting may be normal. All vaginal bleeding during pregnancy should be assessed by a physician, and a large amount of bleeding may indicate a medical emergency. "Bloody show" near term may indicate that delivery is near. Prehospital: Use standard precautions, and position the patient on her left side. Place a sanitary pad over the vaginal opening, and save any soaked pads in a plastic bag so the physician can estimate the amount of blood loss. Manage the patient's airway/ventilation/oxygen supplementation, and provide emotional support. Provide an IV access line and fluids if indicated.

Spontaneous and Elective Abortion and Ectopic Pregnancy

Spontaneous abortion: Unplanned loss of pregnancy at or before 20 weeks. May result from trauma, fetal abnormality, or another cause. Indications include vaginal bleeding (mild to severe) and contractions. The patient may be very emotionally upset. Prehospital: Use the term "miscarriage" rather than "abortion," which has negative connotations for many; gather any products of conception in a plastic bag to take to the hospital; provide supportive care; place a sanitary pad over the vagina; and provide reassurance and emotional support.

Elective abortion: Planned loss of pregnancy at or before 20 weeks per surgical procedure or abortion pills (during the first 10 weeks). Patients may develop bleeding after surgery or as the fetus is expelled. Prehospital: Gather any products of conception in a plastic bag to take to the hospital, provide supportive are, place a sanitary pad over the vagina, and provide reassurance and emotional support.

Ectopic pregnancy: Pregnancy in which the egg fertilizes and attaches outside of the uterus (usually in the fallopian tubes), resulting in abdominal pain, absent menstrual periods, and vaginal bleeding. Prehospital: As above.

Delivery of a Newborn

If the fetal head is obvious at the vaginal opening (crowning), **delivery** is imminent. Steps to delivery include the following:

- Wash hands and don PPE for standard precautions and obtain an OB kit and supplies.
- Position the patient on her back with hips elevated, knees bent, and legs apart.
- Position one person at the mother's head for support if possible while the other supports the baby's head during delivery.
- Provide oxygen to the mother.
- If the umbilical cord is around the baby's neck, attempt to slip it over the infant's head.
- Make note of the time of delivery.
- Lower the infant's head to facilitate drainage of fluids, and keep the mouth and nose suctioned with a bulb syringe.
- Clamp the cord or cut it if sterile equipment is available.

- Monitor the infant's airway, breathing, and circulation with the baby at the level of the birth canal.
- Monitor delivery of the placenta (afterbirth).
- If mother and infant are stable, allow the infant to nurse.
- Place a sanitary pad over the vaginal opening to contain any bleeding. Observe for hemorrhage.
- Massage the uterus in a circular motion to prevent excessive bleeding.

Complications of Pregnancy and Labor

Complication	Characteristic	Prehospital
Preterm labor	Labor between weeks 20 and 37; presents a risk to the fetus.	Provide supportive care. Manage the patient's airway/ventilation/ oxygen supplementation (100%). Transport rapidly if there is severe bleeding or a risk of imminent preterm delivery.
Premature rupture of membranes	Membranes rupture before the onset of labor; this may lead to preterm labor and risk to the fetus.	
Substance abuse	May result in damage to the fetus and preterm labor. Many drugs restrict blood flow to the fetus, resulting in growth retardation and low oxygen. Some drugs, such as cocaine, affect the fetal nervous system. Sudden withdrawal of opiates may trigger preterm labor. Alcohol may result in fetal alcohol syndrome, characterized by facial abnormalities, growth retardation, and neurological defects.	
Placental abruption	The placenta prematurely detaches, partially or completely, from the uterus. Related to maternal hypertension, and the incidence increases with cocaine abuse. Partial detachment interferes with the functioning of the placenta, causing intrauterine growth retardation. Severe bleeding occurs with total detachment.	
Placenta previa	Placenta implants over or near the internal cervical opening. Implantation may be complete (covering the entire opening), partial, or marginal (to the edge of the cervical opening). Results in increased incidences of hemorrhage in the third trimester. Symptoms include painless bleeding after the 20th week of gestation.	Provide supportive care. Manage the patient's airway/ventilation/o xygen supplementation (100%). Transport rapidly if there is severe bleeding, high BP ≥160/110, seizures, or altered mental status.
Pregnancy-induced hypertension/ Preeclampsia/ Eclampsia	Hypertension >140/90 associated with increased protein in the urine and edema (peripheral or generalized) or an increase of ≥5 pounds of weight in one week after the 20th week of gestation. Severe preeclampsia is BP ≥160/110. Symptoms include headache, abdominal pain, and visual disturbances. May progress to eclampsia (seizures) and death.	

Complications of Delivery

Complication	Characteristic	Prehospital
Cephalic (vertex) presentation	Military: Head straight, neck not flexed. Brow: Neck extended, brow presents first, can cause birth trauma so episiotomy or cesarean section (C-section) is usually required. Face: Severely extended neck with face presentation, may prolong labor, increase swelling of the fetus, and cause neck trauma.	Provide supportive care. Manage the patient's airway/ventilation/ oxygen supplementation (100%). Transport rapidly.
Breech presentation	Frank breech (buttocks presentation with legs extended upward) is the most common, but single- or double-footling breech (incomplete breech) or buttocks presentation with legs flexed (complete breech) can also occur. Breech presentation is most common with placenta previa, hydramnios, fetal anomalies, and multiple gestations. Cord prolapse is more likely. Head trauma may occur because molding does not occur, and the head can become entrapped.	

Prolapse of the Umbilical Cord

A **prolapse of the umbilical cord** occurs when the umbilical cord precedes the fetus in the birth canal and becomes entrapped by the descending fetus. With an occult cord prolapse, the umbilical cord is beside or just ahead of the fetal head. With a nuchal cord prolapse, the cord tightly wraps about the fetal neck. About half of prolapses occur in the second stage of labor and relate to premature delivery, multiple gestations, or other complications. As contractions occur and the head descends, pressure to the umbilical cord occludes the blood flow, causing hypoxia and bradycardia. The decrease in blood flow through the umbilical vessels can cause impaired gas exchange, and if pressure on the cord is not relieved, the fetus can suffer severe neurological damage or death. Prehospital: Elevate the presenting part off the cord, slip the cord off of the fetus's neck if possible, elevate the mother's knees to the chest to relieve pressure on the cord, provide 100% oxygen, and transport rapidly.

Initial Care of the Newborn

Dr. Virginia Apgar developed the **APGAR assessment** in 1952. APGAR stands for **a**ppearance, **p**ulse, **g**rimace, **a**ctivity, and **r**espiration. The APGAR is the first test given to a newborn. It is used as a quick evaluation of a newborn's physical condition to determine if any emergency medical care is needed, and it is administered 1 minute and 5 minutes after birth. The test is administered more than once because the baby's condition may change rapidly. It may be administered for a third time 10 minutes after birth, if needed. The baby is rated on the five subscales, and the scores are added together. A total score of ≥7 is a sign of good health.

APGAR Assessment

Sign	0	1	2
Appearance (skin color)	Cyanotic or pallor over entire body	Normal, except for the extremities	Entire body is normal.
Pulse (heart rate)	Absent	<100 bpm	>100 bpm.
Grimace (reflex irritability)	Unresponsive	Grimace	Infant sneezes, coughs, and recoils.
Activity (muscle tone)	Absent	Flexed limbs	Infant moves freely.
Respiration (breathing rate and effort)	Absent	Bradypnea, dyspnea	Good breathing and crying.

Routine Care of the Newborn

The infant should be given a **rapid assessment** within seconds of birth to determine if he or she is at term, if the amniotic fluid is clear, if there is muscle tone, and if there are respirations or crying. If any of these conditions are not met, then further resuscitation is needed. The basic steps to care include the following:

- Warming the infant after drying.
- Positioning the infant and clearing the airway if necessary.
- Stimulating and repositioning the infant.

The child should be evaluated throughout the initial procedures as follows:

- Respirations: The rate and character of the respirations should be noted as well as an observation of chest wall movement.
- Heart rate: Should be >100 bpm, assessed with a stethoscope or at the base of the umbilical cord.

Infants have poor temperature regulation ability, particularly preterm infants who lack brown fat, which is one of the body's tools to regulate body temperature, so **providing warmth** is critical as a component of resuscitation. An infant who is just seconds old and wet will need aggressive measures to keep him or her warm while any resuscitation efforts are being initiated. Infants lose heat through their heads, so one of the first steps should be to place a hat on the head or cover the head in some way. The infant should be vigorously dried with warmed blankets. Often, this stimulation—drying and warming—is all that is needed to establish a regular respiration pattern in the neonate. Preterm infants weighing <1500 grams should be placed in a plastic bag (made specifically for this purpose), if available, up to the height of the shoulders to prevent cold shock. A term infant with no apparent distress can be placed on the mother's chest and covered with a warm blanket.

To **establish an airway**, the infant is placed supine with the head slightly extended in the "sniffing" position. A small neck roll may be placed under the shoulders to maintain this position in a very small premature infant. Once the proper position is established, the mouth and nose are suctioned (suction the mouth first to prevent reflex inspiration of secretions when the nose is suctioned) with a bulb syringe or catheter if necessary. The infant's head can be turned momentarily to the side to allow secretions to pool in the cheek where they can be more easily suctioned and removed to establish the airway. **Stimulating** the newborn is often all that is needed to initiate spontaneous respirations. This tactile stimulation can be accomplished by gently rubbing the back or trunk of the

- 115 -

infant. Another technique that is used to provide stimulation is flicking or rubbing the soles of the feet. Slapping neonates as stimulation is no longer practiced and should NOT be used.

Pediatric Considerations

Pediatric patients have the following general considerations:

- Proportionately greater body surface area to body mass ratio, so they are at greater risk of fluid and heat loss, burns, and absorption of toxins.
- Higher respiratory rates and heart rates than adults, resulting in higher oxygen demand.
- Immature blood/brain barrier, resulting in more neurological symptoms.
- Immature immune system, resulting in a higher risk of infection.
- Narrower and shorter airway and smaller jaw, so the tongue may easily obstruct the airway.
- Soft tracheal cartilage that increases the risk of airway collapse, large epiglottis.
- More pliable ribs, which provide less protection for abdominal organs, which are more forward.
- Liver and spleen that are proportionately larger and at risk of injury.
- Bones that are softer with open growth plates: An open growth plate injury can impair growth.
- Less protection for the brain and spinal cord (increasing the risk of injury) and less subarachnoid space.
- Cerebral blood-flow needs twice that of adults, increasing the risk of hypoxia.
- Limited glucose stores and risk of hypothermia (especially in the first month).
- Anterior fontanel that closes by 12 months and posterior fontanel that closes by 3–4 months.

Pediatric Assessment

Pediatric assessment should include the following:

- Pediatric assessment triangle:
  - Appearance (abnormal tone, decreased interactivity, decreased consolability, abnormal look/gaze, and abnormal speech or cry).
  - Work of breathing (abnormal sounds [wheezing, stridor], position, retractions [sternum], flaring [nostrils], and apnea/gasping).
  - Circulation (pallor, mottling, and cyanosis).
- Assess airway, breathing, and circulation (heart rate/pulse): Place in the shock position and provide a warming blanket for signs of shock.
- Ventilation/oxygenation: Administer oxygen and assist with ventilation if it is abnormal.
- Determine the patient's level of consciousness: Use the alert, voice, pain, unresponsive (AVPU) assessment. Note movement of the extremities and whether the pupils are normal, dilated, constricted, reactive, or fixed.
- Prevent hypothermia: Cover with a warming blanket, cover the head, and avoid unnecessary exposure of the skin.
- Obtain the medical history from the caregiver/parent: Include the type and duration of symptoms, fever, level of activity, recent foods/fluids, medications, medication allergies, past or chronic illnesses, and events leading to the current problem.
- Head-to-toe physical examination: Note any bruising, swelling, drainage, loose teeth, unusual odors, bleeding, rashes, deformities, and pain on movement.

- 116 -

Pediatric Seizures

Febrile seizure is a generalized seizure associated with fever (usually >38.8°C [101.8°F]) from any type of infection (upper respiratory, urinary tract) but without intracranial infection or other cause, occurring between 6 months and 5 years of age. Seizures usually last <15 minutes and are without subsequent neurological deficit. Prehospital: Provide fever control (acetaminophen OR ibuprofen) and a tepid-water bath.

Other types of seizures may result from pathology, such as meningitis, cerebral edema, brain trauma, or brain tumors, but most seizures in children >3 are related to idiopathic epilepsy, which predisposes the child to recurrent seizures, usually of the same type. Seizures are characterized as focal (localized), focal with rapid generalization (spreading), and generalized (widespread). In most children, seizures become generalized with loss of consciousness. Seizure disorders with onset younger than 4 years of age usually cause more neurological damage than those with onset at older than 4 years of age. Prehospital: Place the patient on the floor or on a safe surface, loosen clothes, and protect him or her from injury during seizure. Afterwards, place the patient in the recovery position, monitor the airway/ventilation, and provide oxygen supplementation (the patient may need assisted ventilation if he or she is cyanotic) and suction if needed.

Growth and Development of Pediatric Patients

Age	Characteristics
0–2 mos.	Sleeps up to 16 hours a day but should rouse easily. Cries for a reason; persistent crying may indicate illness. Limited head control. Gazes at faces.
2–6 mos.	Smiles voluntarily and makes eye contact, uses both hands, begins to hold head up, rolls over, and sleeps through the night.
6–12 mos.	Sits, crawls, has pincer grasp, mouths objects (increasing risk of poisoning and aspiration), babbles, and speaks first words by 12 months. Exhibits separation anxiety from parents.
12–18 mos.	Begins to walk; imitates others; knows body parts and 4–6 words; lacks molars for grinding food, increasing the risk of aspiration; and has increased mobility.
18–24 mos.	Begins to run and climb, knows 100 words (24 months), clings to parents, attaches to special objects, labels objects, and begins to understand cause and effect.
2–5 years	Walks, runs, throws, catches, is toilet trained, has magical thinking and irrational fears, learns acceptable behavior, has temper tantrums, and develops modesty.
6–12 years	Loses baby teeth; thinks logically; becomes self-conscious; understand the finality of death; attaches importance to school, popularity, and peers.
12–20 years	Puberty begins, reasons (imperfectly), is self-conscious, seeks independence and peer approval, and takes risks.

Apparent Life-Threatening Events (ALTEs) and Sudden Infant Death Syndrome (SIDS)

Infants with an **apparent life-threatening event (ALTE)** are those who are lifeless and without respirations but are successfully resuscitated or begin breathing spontaneously. With **sudden infant death syndrome (SIDS),** which is almost always related to respiratory arrest, the child cannot be resuscitated. There are numerous proposed causes for ALTE and SIDS, so a careful history, including familial history of SIDS, and physical examination or postmortem examination can provide important information, such as indications of child abuse or metabolic/infectious disorders. Prehospital: Continue resuscitative efforts (airway/ventilation/oxygen supplementation, compressions as indicated) and stabilize the infant if possible. The child with ALTE should be hospitalized for observation, further studies, and apnea monitoring because these children are at an increased risk for SIDS. For SIDS patients, the paramedic should provide support and information to the family. The protocol for reporting SIDS varies by state, but it usually involves notifying the coroner's office.

Geriatric Considerations

Geriatric patients may have the following considerations:

- Decreased sensory input (hearing, vision, touch, pain); impaired depth perception and night vision; and decreased ability to differentiate colors.
- Hypertension, increasing the risk of heart attack and stroke.
- Decreased breathing capacity and decreased cough, increasing the risk of infection.
- Difficulty chewing and swallowing; digestive problems; and reflux when lying flat, increasing the risk of aspiration.
- Short-term memory deficit and slower reflexes.
- Decreased bone density, increasing the risk of breaks; loss of muscle tone.
- Increased risk of infection and less obvious symptoms of infection.
- Arthritis in the neck, interfering with airway assessment.
- Dentures that can obstruct the airway (leave them in place if possible during ventilation).
- Skin that is fragile and tears easily.
- Irregular pulse from underlying heart problems.
- Dementia (incidence increases with age), making history taking and treatment difficult.
- Atypical symptoms for illnesses, even if severely ill.
- Multiple comorbidities and multiple medications.
- Shock with BP greater than 100.

Delirium

Delirium is an acute sudden change in consciousness, characterized by reduced ability to focus or sustain attention, language and memory disturbance, disorientation, confusion, audiovisual hallucinations, sleep disturbance, and psychomotor activity disorder. Delirium differs from disorders with similar symptoms in that delirium is fluctuating. Delirium occurs in 10%–40% of hospitalized older adults and about 80% of patients who are terminally ill. Delirium may result from drugs such as anticholinergics and numerous conditions including infection, hypoxia, trauma, dementia, depression, vision and hearing loss, surgery, alcoholism, untreated pain, fluid/electrolyte imbalance, and malnutrition. Delirium increases the risks of morbidity and death, especially if untreated. Asking the patient to count backward from 20 to 1 and spell his or her first name backward can identify an attention deficit. Prehospital: Ensure the patient's safety, manage the patient's airway/ventilation/oxygen supplementation, and reorient the patient frequently.

Heart Failure

Heart failure (HF, aka congestive HF) includes disorders of contractions (systolic "left-sided" dysfunction) or filling (diastolic dysfunction) or both, which result in hypertrophy (thickening, enlarging, and stiffening) of the myocardium (heart muscle). The most common causes are coronary artery disease, myocardial infarction, systemic or pulmonary hypertension, cardiomyopathy, and valvular disorders. Incidence of HF correlates with age. Left-sided HF may cause pulmonary edema that impairs ventilation, leading to hypoxia, especially when the patient is lying in a supine position, and right-sided HF may cause abdominal and peripheral edema of the feet and legs. The circulatory time with HF decreases overall, so changes in oximetry to show hypoxia may be delayed. The autonomic nervous system's regulation of breathing to control oxygen levels may be impaired, resulting in periodic breathing patterns, Cheyne-Stokes breathing, or central sleep apnea. Medications used to treat HF include ACE inhibitors (captopril, lisinopril), angiotensin receptor blockers (ARBs) (losartan, valsartan), beta-blockers (metoprolol, carvedilol), aldosterone agonists (spironolactone), and diuretics (hydrochlorothiazide, furosemide).

Chronic Versus Acute Heart Failure

Chronic heart failure develops insidiously over time as the heart muscles weaken and enlarge, so initially patients may only note fatigue, weight gain, and swelling in their feet and ankles. **Acute heart failure** is characterized by impairment of gas exchange and decreased cardiac output because of changes in preload, contractibility, and heart rhythm; symptoms are more acute and may include irregular heartbeat, chest pain, cough, and rapid breathing, wheezing, and cyanosis from lack of adequate oxygen. Patients may also suffer from anxiety, decreased activity tolerance, and disturbances in sleep patterns. Medical management is aimed at increasing cardiac function, providing support, and monitoring treatment. Patients often are acutely short of breath and sitting upright, with rales evident in their lungs. Assessment includes conducting primary and secondary surveys; taking a complete medical history including medication use/home oxygen use; and assessing the patient's level of consciousness, airway status (cough, sputum, labored breathing, tripod position), heart rate/rhythm, peripheral pulses, edema (pitting/nonpitting, ascites, sacral), and complications. Prehospital: Manage the patient's airway/ventilation/oxygen supplementation with a nonrebreather mask or BVM with high-flow oxygen, position for comfort, and suction if necessary.

Thromboembolism and Pulmonary Embolism

Thromboembolism includes the formation of a thrombus (such as in the heart with atrial fibrillation and in the deep veins with immobilization) and an embolism in which a clot breaks off and travels through the circulatory system. Although thromboembolism may cause a heart attack or stroke, the most common presentation is a **pulmonary embolism (PE)** resulting from deep vein thrombosis. The patient may or may not complain of pain at the thrombus site, which may be swollen and erythematous (red), typically in a lower extremity. When the patient develops PE, the usual presentation is acute onset of dyspnea and tachycardia and sitting in the tripod position. Some patients may have ECG abnormalities, frothy sputum, cough, fever, hemoptysis, and jugular vein distension. Prehospital: Provide supportive care; manage the patient's airway/ventilation/intubation as needed with oxygen to maintain oxygen saturation >94%.

Dementia

Type of dementia	Characteristics
Alzheimer's	Progressive dementia beginning with short-term memory loss and difficulty remembering names. It progresses to impaired judgment; disorientation; confusion; behavioral changes; difficulty understanding, reading, and using language; dysphagia; incoordination and inability to walk; and incontinence.
Creutzfeldt-Jakob disease	Rapidly progressive prion disease with impaired memory, behavioral changes, and incoordination, leading to death.
Huntington's disease	Progressive genetic disorder characterized by involuntary movements, muscle rigidity, abnormal eye movement, ataxia, lack of impulse and behavioral control, increasing confusion, difficulty communicating, and depression.
Pick's disease (frontotemporal dementia)	Form of progressive dementia resulting in destruction of neurons with change of personality and lack of judgment and empathy. Loss of language may include ability to understand and communicate.
Wernicke's encephalopathy	Inflammatory hemorrhagic encephalopathy due to thiamine deficiency, often associated with alcoholism. Symptoms include paralyzed eye muscles; double vision; ataxia; and a range of mental changes from forgetfulness to delirium tremens and Korsakoff's psychosis, which can lead to amnesia, disorientation, and hallucinations. Patients are able to produce language, although with some impairment, such as incorrect words or sounds, but they may have difficulty understanding.

Elder Abuse

Physical	Various types of assault related to hitting, kicking, pulling hair, shoving, and pushing. Patients may be forcibly confined, forced into seclusion, and/or force-fed to the point that they choke on food.
Psychological	Caregivers may threaten to hit the patient, brandish a weapon, and/or tell the person to commit suicide. Ongoing intimidation may make the patient terrified and anxious. Sometimes, caregivers threaten to injure pets or family members, increasing the patient's fear.
Sexual	Types of sexual abuse include the following: Physical: Fondling, kissing, and rape. Emotional: Exhibitionism. Verbal: Sexual harassment, using obscene language, and threatening.
Financial	Financial abuse includes the following: Outright stealing of property or persuading patients to give away possessions. Forcing patients to sign away property. Emptying bank and savings accounts and using stolen credit cards. Convincing the person to invest money in fraudulent schemes. Taking money for home renovations that are not done.

Child Abuse

Children rarely admit to **abuse** (physical, sexual, or emotional) and often attempt to protect the abusing parent. Therefore, suspicion of abuse depends on other indicators such as the following:

- **Behavioral:** The child may be overly compliant or fearful with obvious changes in demeanor when a parent/caregiver is present. Some children act out with aggression toward other children or animals. Children may become depressed or suicidal or present with sleeping or eating disorders. Behaviors may become increasingly self-destructive as the child ages, including inappropriate sexualized behavior.
- **Physical/Sexual:** The type, location, and extent of injuries can raise the suspicion of abuse. Head and facial injuries and bruising are common, as are bite or burn marks and spiral fractures. There may be handprints or grab marks and unusual bruising, such as across the buttocks. Any bruising, swelling, or tearing of the genital area and the identification of sexually transmitted diseases are also causes for concern.

Suspected abuse must be reported to the appropriate authorities, according to protocol, with careful documentation of findings and statements by the child or caregivers.

Neglect and Lack of Supervised Care

Children and older or impaired adults may suffer from profound **neglect or a lack of supervision** that places them at risk. Indicators include the following:

- Appearing dirty and unkempt, sometimes with infestations of lice, and wearing ill-fitting, torn clothing and shoes.
- Being tired and sleepy during the daytime.
- Having excessive medical or dental problems, such as extensive dental caries.
- Missing doctor appointments and not receiving proper immunizations.
- Being underweight for their current stage of development.
- Lacking assistive devices or misplaced hearing aids/eyeglasses.
- Left in soiled or urine-/feces-soiled clothing.
- Clothing is inadequate (such as lack of a coat/sweater during winter or dirty, torn, ill-fitting clothes).

Neglect can be difficult to assess, especially if the EMT is serving a homeless or very disadvantaged population. Home visits may be needed to ascertain if there is adequate food, clothing, or supervision, and this is beyond the scope of care provided by the EMT. Thus, suspicions should be reported to the appropriate authorities who can arrange a follow-up assessment of the home environment.

Injuries Consistent with Domestic Violence/Abuse

Characteristic injuries	Ruptured eardrum. Rectal/genital injury—burns, bites, trauma. Scrapes and bruises about the neck, face, head, trunk, arms. Cuts, bruises, and fractures of the face.
Patterns of injuries	"Bathing suit" pattern—injuries on parts of body that are usually covered with clothing because the perpetrator wants to hide the evidence of abuse. Head and neck injuries (50%).
Abusive injuries (rarely attributable to accidents)	Bites, bruises, rope and cigarette burns, and welts in the outline of weapons (belt marks). Bilateral injuries of the arms/legs.
Defensive injuries	Back-of-the-body injury from being attacked while crouched on the floor facedown. Located on the soles of the feet from kicking at a perpetrator. Located on the ulnar aspect of the hands or palm from blocking blows.

Patients with Special Challenges

Condition	Issues	Prehospital considerations
Homeless/ Indigent	Patients often are without medical care, increasing the risk of disease, and they may lack insurance. They may have mental health/substance abuse problems.	Know who will treat indigent patients and what resources are available in the community.
Bariatric	Increased risk of chronic disease. Patients pose handling/moving problems and require special bariatric equipment and multiple personnel to assist. Patients often have trouble breathing and must have their head elevated.	Recognize the need for bariatric equipment and know how/where to obtain it. Notify the receiving facility. Use properly sized equipment, such as BP cuffs.
Technology-/Device-assisted	Wide range of issues including ventilators, apnea monitors, vascular devices, dialysis shunts, colostomies, ileostomies, and feeding tubes. Patients may have special needs regarding care and transport.	Ask about the patient's equipment and needs. Avoid disturbing/damaging the devices if possible.

EMS Operations

Apparatus and Equipment Readiness

The EMT should ensure that the ambulance is ready for use and that the tires are properly inflated, the gas tank is full, warning devices are working, and engine fluid levels are appropriate. All necessary safety equipment, such as PPE (masks, gowns, gloves, and goggles or face guards) and safety devices (safety vests, road flares, and signs) as well as seat belts and harnesses, should be available and in proper working condition. All equipment in the cab, the compartments, and the rear of the ambulance should be in the proper place, labeled, and secured to prevent shifting during transportation. High-risk situations include going through intersections, inclement weather (especially with poor visibility), careless drivers, highway access, unpaved roads, and driver distractions (conversation, eating, drinking, mobile devices, music, GPS devices, and fatigue). During transportation, all personnel as well as patients should be properly secured with safety equipment.

Scene-of-Incident Safety Considerations

The EMT must do a 360° **assessment of the scene** of incident on arrival and determine safety considerations. The EMT should make note of any gunshots heard, downed power lines, buildings in a state of collapse, leaking fuels/fluids, fire, smoke, broken glass, and other hazards. The EMT may need to wait until the site is safe to proceed. The EMT should assess the mechanism of injury (accidents) and the need for appropriate PPE (gloves, gown, mask, face guard) and must keep the patient informed of all actions and prevent harm or further injury. The ambulance should be parked off of the roadway if possible or parked at a 45° angle (front wheels out) to shield the work area, making sure not to block access for other emergency vehicles. Parking uphill is safer than downhill and upwind rather than downwind. If flares are used to warn other drivers, they should extend at least 300 feet from a collision. Yellow warning lights at the scene are the safest, but excessive lighting may blind other drivers at night.

Transferring a Patient from the Scene to an Ambulance

Different types of **stretchers** and **transfer equipment** may be used for prehospital transfer, including the following:

- Wheeled: Stretcher that can be lowered and raised with a wheeled base allowing it to slide into the ambulance.
- Scoop: Two- to four-piece stretcher that can be connected and placed under a patient.
- Transfer sheet: A heavy plastic sheet can be used with patients up to 800 lb to facilitate transfer.
- Flexible stretcher: Lightweight flexible (plastic, rubberized canvas) stretcher with webbing handles on both sides. Can be used to transfer patients around corners and up and down stairs where a wheeled stretcher cannot be used.
- Stair chair: Safety chair that can be used to transfer patients in tight spaces and up and down stairs.
- Lightweight stretcher: Folding stretcher made of lightweight materials.
- Basket stretcher (Stokes basket): Used primarily for rescues in the wilderness or from cliffs.

Patient positioning should be according to the possible or probable injury, with safety restraints always securing the patient to the gurney and the gurney to the vehicle.

- <u>Left-side-lying</u>: Pregnant patients should be placed in this position to increase circulation to the placenta, and unconscious patients should be placed in this position to prevent aspiration and choking if there is no indication of a spinal injury.
- <u>Supine</u> (flat on the back): Patient has a suspected pelvic fracture or neck injury (also requires a cervical collar).
- <u>Supine</u> (feet elevated above the heart): This is the position for patients in shock to increase circulation to the heart and brain as the BP falls.
- <u>Trendelenburg</u> (the entire stretcher is tilted so that the head is below the feet): Position for patients with a suspected spinal cord injury.
- <u>Semi-Fowler's</u> (30- to 45-degree position): For patients with chest pain, stroke, and/or shortness of breath and no indication of a spinal cord injury.
- <u>Fowler's</u> (upright, 90-degree position): For patients with severe shortness of breath.

Environmental Risk Factors

When assessing a patient, it's important to consider that **environmental factors** may place the patient at an increased risk for harm or may be a factor in disease. There are a number of different types of environmental factors to consider.

Factors	Examples	Effects
Toxic chemicals	Lead, arsenic, muriatic acid, sulfuric acid, ammonia, lime	May result in poisoning (lead, arsenic) or burns (acids, ammonia, lime) through direct exposure or inhalation
Physical objects	Guns, cars, knives, equipment	Accidents, gunshot wounds, stabbings, various injuries (blunt and penetrating)
Biological organisms	Bacteria, fungi, viruses	Infections
Temperature variations	Heat, cold	Burns, dehydration, heat stroke, hyperthermia, hypothermia, frostbite
Ambient noise	Sirens, loud music, traffic noise, work-related noise	Hearing loss/deafness, increased anxiety
Psychosocial	Increased stress	Anxiety, hypertension, suicidal ideation

Rescues in Confined Spaces

A **confined space** is one in which access is limited and the space is surrounded by walls or structures that are not suitable for habitation. A confined space may occur in a building (such as with a collapse), a silo, a motor vehicle (such as a large vehicle involved in a crash), a cistern or septic tank, or a well. A confined space may pose a risk to the patient and the EMT because of difficulty moving about and accessing the patient as well as decreased ventilation that may result in the buildup of toxic gases and/or a lack of oxygen. Before entering a confined space, the EMT should test the atmosphere and use the correct breathing equipment. This is especially important if the patient is nonresponsive, which is often an indication of poor air quality. The EMT should also carefully assess his or her ability to access the patient and the best means of doing so.

Driving Safety

The **ambulance driver** should stop briefly or slow significantly at intersections because other drivers may not hear or may ignore sirens. The driver should keep the brake covered with the left foot for fast braking and avoid excessive speeds because of the increased risk of accidents, especially on curves. The speed should be adjusted for road and weather conditions and should not be influenced by use of the siren (siren syndrome). Snow and ice should be cleared from the ambulance before driving it. At least one vehicle length should separate the ambulance from other vehicles for every 10 mph of speed. A spotter should always be used when backing up the ambulance because of poor visibility. All personnel in the ambulance should be seated and secured with seat belts or safety harnesses before the ambulance moves. Studies have shown that CPR is most effective if done from a sitting position in an ambulance rather than standing, despite common practice. Patients and gurneys should also be secured.

Lights and Sirens

Lights and sirens should be used together, and they are indicated when going to a scene and when transporting a patient in a serious emergent situation. There are four types of warning lights used on emergency vehicles such as ambulances: rotating lights (resulting in a flashing sensation), fixed flashes (usually red or blue), strobe lights, and LED lights. Red (the most common) and blue lights are generally used to indicate emergency vehicles and can be used to obtain the right-of-way or to block the right-of-way. These colors may be interchangeable, although in some states the color blue is restricted to law enforcement vehicles. Amber lights are warning lights and can be used by all vehicles, but they do not require others to stop. Some emergency vehicle lights change to amber when the vehicle is parked. White warning lights cannot be used on the rear of an emergency vehicle. Green lights are sometimes used to indicate a mobile incident command post, but in some states, green lights may also indicate private security vehicles or volunteer firefighters.

Incident Management

FEMA IS-700.A NIMS

FEMA IS-700.A outlines the **National Incident Management System (NIMS)**, which, under the direction of the Federal Emergency Management Agency (FEMA), an agency of the U.S. Department of Homeland Security, provides the foundation for collaboration among different governmental and nongovernmental agencies, jurisdictions, and specialties/disciplines in handling large-scale incidents that threaten life, property, and/or the environment. Components of FEMA IS-700.A include the following:

- Preparedness: Focuses on planning, procedures and protocols, training and exercises, personnel qualifications/certification, and equipment certification, and it includes the National Response Framework, which ensures that local jurisdictions retain control but use a unified approach and establishes protocols.
- Communications and information management: Systems must be interoperable, reliable, portable, scalable, resilient, and redundant.
- Resource management: Includes personnel, equipment, supplies, and facilities, which must be inventoried and categorized using a standardized approach.
- Command and management: Includes the Incident Command System (this standardized approach outlines the responsibilities of the incident commander, area command, command staff, and general staff), multiagency coordination systems, and public information.
- Management and maintenance: The National Integration Center (NIC) is responsible for NIMS management.
- Flexibility: Components are scalable and adaptable to all types of incidents.
- Standardization: The NIC develops standards in cooperation with standards development organizations.

ICS-100.B

ICS-100.B, the **Incident Command System** course, meets NIMS requirements for operational personnel and outlines a standardized approach to incident management. ICS is used for any type of major event, planned or otherwise, and large- or small-scale incidents, including natural (disasters), technological (hazmat release), and human-caused (civil disturbance) hazards. ICS outlines the chain of command (the incident commander in control and orders going through supervisors). Every incident requires an incident action plan, resource management, and processes for reimbursement. The incident commander establishes an incident command post and staging areas (gathering places) as well a base (coordination area for logistic and administrative functions), camps (for sleeping, eating, and sanitary services), helibases, and helispots. Primary features of ICS include common terminology, establishment/transfer of command, chain of command/unity of command, management of objects, incident action planning, modular organization, manageable span of control, comprehensive resource management, incident facilities and locations, integrated communications, information and intelligence management, accountability, and dispatch/deployment.

Chain of Command/Unity of Command/Unified Command

Each organization must establish the **chain of command** for its incident command system. Although these may vary somewhat, an incident commander is ultimately in charge with individuals being assigned as incident managers in different areas, such as triage, treatment, transport, security, and liaison. **Unity of command** means that each incident commander should have control over personnel assigned to his or her area, and each individual within the chain of command should have a clear understanding of whom to report to at the scene so that communication is efficient and timely. **Unified command** means that when multiple agencies are involved from multiple jurisdictions, the chain of command that has been established is recognized and respected even though each agency retains its own authority and accountability and is responsible for carrying out its own duties. A unified command system prevents duplication of effort as well as neglect of important functions.

Incident Action Plan

The purpose of the **incident action plan** is to outline control objectives, resources, and strategies for dealing with an incident. Incident action plans should be updated frequently. Incident action plans may be designed for various types of incidents (terrorist attack, disease outbreak, hurricane) and modified as needed and should include the following:

- Goals and objectives, including expected outcomes.
- Strategies and tactics for responding and accomplishing the goals and objectives.
- An outline of the chain of command for the incident command system, including the span of control (the number of people reporting to an individual).
- Tasks assigned to each level in the chain of command.
- Safety/Health plan for responders to prevent injury/illness and to treat as needed.
- Communications plan outlining how information will be exchanged, including alternative methods of command if, for example, cell phone towers are out of commission.
- Logistics plan regarding the acquisition and use of resources, such as supplies, personnel, and equipment.
- Maps and demographic information.

Incident Commander

When a multiple-casualty or mass-casualty event occurs, the first lead emergency medical responder on the scene generally assumes the role of **incident commander** and carries out a rapid assessment of the scene and begins to call for additional resources as indicated while another medical responder begins triage. The incident commander should begin to establish a command center in an area that is safe and out of the way of emergency vehicles while awaiting assistance. This first incident commander will relinquish the role when the staffed and/or assigned incident commander arrives to take command and should then report to the person who is assuming the role of staging officer. The incident commander's duties include establishing command, assessing needs, developing a plan, coordinating all activities, delegating responsibilities, ensuring the safety of all personnel and patients, liaising with other agencies, and communicating information.

Primary Triage and Resource Management

Primary triage is a rapid method (30–60 seconds) of prioritizing patients based on the severity of their condition, and it is carried out at the scene of multiple-casualty incidents. All patients are triaged and tagged according to the following international color-coding priority (P) guidelines on the foot or wrist (not on the clothing):

- P1—Red: Immediate care is needed for urgent systemic life-threatening conditions, such as airway/breathing problems, severe bleeding, severe burns (especially with breathing problems), decreased mental status, shock, and severe medical problems, or a Glasgow Coma Scale score of ≤13.
- P2—Yellow: Delayed care and able to wait 45–60 minutes for treatment. Conditions include burns (without breathing problems), multiple bone/joint injuries, back and/or spinal cord injuries (unless the patient is in respiratory distress).
- P3—Green: Hold, able to wait hours for treatment of minor injuries.
- P4—Black: Deceased.

Resource management involves identifying a triage officer, who remains at the scene during the event and identifying the need for additional personnel and equipment and providing those to the patients with the highest priority.

Secondary Triage/Retriage

During a mass-casualty incident, triage is done quickly, and patients may be scattered over a wide area with many patients being red-tagged for emergency care. Patients coded black are left in place, but those with other-color tags should be moved and segregated in separate sections of a holding area to await treatment and/or transport. The patients should be **retriaged** as they are moved into the holding area to determine if the tagging color is still appropriate. Additionally, **secondary triage** may be carried out in the separate sections, especially if some must be airlifted, to determine which patients have the best chance of survival and should receive priority for transfer and treatment. Secondary triage may also help to determine which trauma center (based on location or level of care) or hospital is most appropriate for the patient considering the patient's condition, transport time, and the surge capacity of the healthcare institutions.

Centers for Disease Control and Prevention Guidelines for Field Triage of Injured Patients

The **CDC's guidelines for field triage** of injured patients is a four-step algorithm that is used to identify the most seriously ill patients and transport them to an appropriate treatment center.

Step	Assess	Findings requiring priority treatment	Plan
1	Vital signs/Level of consciousness	Glasgow Coma Scale score of ≤13, systolic BP <90 mm Hg, respiratory rate <10 or >29 per minute (<20 in an infant <1 year), or need of ventilatory support.	Highest level trauma center
2	Anatomy of injury	Penetrating injuries, flail chest, two or more long-bone fractures, crushed/mangled/pulseless extremity, amputations, pelvic fractures, open/depressed skull fracture, or paralysis.	Highest level trauma center
3	Mechanism of injury/High-energy impact	Falls—adults >20 feet and children >10 feet or 2–3 times their height. High-risk auto crash with intrusions, partial or complete ejection, or there is a death in the same passenger compartment. Auto vs. pedestrian/bicycle with victim thrown, run over, or sustaining a significant impact. Motorcycle crash >20 mph.	Trauma center
4	Special patient/system considerations	Older adults, children, pregnancy >30 weeks, burns, patients on anticoagulants or with bleeding disorders (based on the EMT's best judgment).	Trauma center/Hospital

START Method of Triage

With the **START method of triage**, the paramedic starts triage with the first victim encountered, tags the patient, and then moves to the next patient, assessing in order: (1) respirations, (2) perfusion, and (3) mental status (RPM) and using the standard red-yellow-green-black color-coding system. Walking wounded are tagged as green.

Respirations	Present.	Red tag if >30. Continue to perfusion assessment if <30.
	Not present—position the airway.	Red tag if respirations recur or black tag (death) if none.
Perfusion	Radial pulse absent or capillary refill of greater than 2 seconds.	Control bleeding and red tag.
	Radial pulse present and capillary refill time of less than 2 seconds.	Continue to mental status assessment.
Mental status	Cannot follow simple directions.	Red tag.
	Can follow simple directions.	Yellow tag.

JumpSTART Method of Triage for Pediatric Patients

JumpSTART is a pediatric triage method developed only for use in multiple-casualty incidents.

Able to walk	No	Continue to breathing assessment.
	Yes	Green tag. Carry out secondary triage.
Breathing	No	Step 1: Position upper airway and red tag if breathing. Step 2: Give five rescue breaths and red tag if breathing. Black tag if breathing does not recur.
	Yes	Respiratory rate <15 or >45, red tag. Respiratory rate 15 to 45, continue to pulse assessment.
Palpable pulse	No	Red tag.
	Yes	Continue to AVPU assessment.
Alert, voice, pain, unresponsive (AVPU) assessment	Inappropriate pain, posturing, or unresponsive	Red tag.
	A, V, or P is appropriate	Yellow tag.

Critical Incident Stress Management (CISM)

Critical incident stress management (CISM) is a procedure to help people cope with stressful events, such as disasters, in order to reduce the incidence of post-traumatic stress syndrome (PTSS).

- Defusing sessions usually occur very early, sometimes during or immediately after a stressful event, and they are used to educate personnel who are actively involved about what to expect over the next few days and to provide guidance in handling their feelings and stress levels.
- Debriefing sessions usually follow in one to three days and may be repeated periodically as needed. These sessions may include people who were directly involved as well as those who were indirectly involved. People are encouraged to express their emotions about the event. Critiquing the event or attempting to place blame is not productive as part of the CISM process.
- Follow-up is done at the end of the process, usually after about week, but this time frame can vary.

Air Medical Transport

Air medical transport is indicated when the patient is in need of a high level of care that may be available on an aircraft but not an ambulance, when the patient's condition and need for treatment are time critical, when the patient is located in a remote area where access by ambulance is difficult or would be delayed (helicopter), or when local medical services have exceeded their capacity. Helipads are often available at large hospitals, so the patient can be treated immediately after arrival. Some disadvantages include inclement weather (which may interfere with flight plans) as well as altitude and airspeed limitations. Depending on the aircraft, the cabin size may be inadequate for the patient, personnel, and equipment. Difficult terrain, such as forested or hilly areas may not provide an adequate landing site. Cost is the biggest difference between ground and air transport with air transport often costing tens of thousands of dollars with only part, or in some cases none, of the costs being covered by insurance.

Helicopters have the advantage over fixed-wing aircraft of being able to load a patient at or near the scene rather than having to transport the patient by ambulance to an airport. A paved surface is not necessary for a helicopter landing site, but level grassy or paved sites are preferred, ideally with 100 × 100 feet of clear space, but a minimum area of 60 × 60 feet may be used. Additionally, the area should be free of debris that may be disrupted by the rotor blades and should be clear of structures that may interfere with the aircraft, such as power poles, tall trees, power lines, cables, and antennas. A rotor aircraft does not require that people approach in a crouching position, but people should avoid holding anything over their heads and should generally approach from the front of the aircraft and avoid the rear of the aircraft and the rear rotors.

The pilot in command (PIC) of rotorcraft and fixed-wing aircraft is responsible for the **safety** of the aircraft, crew, emergency medical personnel, and the patient. As with all takeoffs and landings, medical staff and crew must be seated and secured by seat belts. Helmets should be in place and secure. Patients who are violent, confused, or combative should be physically restrained for transport and may also require chemical restraints to ensure their own personal safety as well as the safety of the medical and flight crew. Patients should be offloaded ONLY when a crew member signals the receiving medical personnel to approach the aircraft. With high-altitude fixed-wing air transports, cabins are pressurized but only to the equivalent of 6000–8000 feet, not to sea level. Rotorcraft are usually used to transfer a patient from the scene of an incident to a primary care facility or from the primary care facility to another type of facility, whereas a fixed-wing aircraft is usually used from one facility to another over longer distances.

Communication Issues Associated with Air Medical Services

A **communication specialist** should coordinate all air medical services, including communications within an agency and between agencies regarding all aspects of transport. The communication specialist should have radio communication skills and knowledge of medical terminology, including knowledge of how to obtain information about a patient, navigation, map usage, customer service, weather, aircraft emergencies, as well as FAA and Federal Communications Commission (FCC) regulations that relate to air medical transport. The communication specialist should be familiar with radio frequencies used by EMS. The dispatcher determines whether an aircraft should take off. The communication center may be located in a medical facility, airport, or other space, but it should be free of distractions and have emergency backup electrical power. All air medical transport team members should have knowledge of the radio communication system. Some systems include radio or radio-phone communication, and some systems require the team members to carry pagers, such as two-way satellite pagers. All incoming and outgoing communication should be recorded.

State and Federal Regulations Regarding Air Medical Services

State **statutes** require that aircraft used for air ambulance service must be licensed to provide that service, and the service must ensure that all required medical equipment is available. Although statutes may vary slightly from one state to another, most require that the service be able to provide basic and advanced life support and should provide patients with a description of services and costs. Additionally, the aircraft and crew must comply with Federal Aviation Administration (FAA) regulations and carry insurance to cover injuries that may occur in transport. The FAA carries out periodic inspections of aircraft and issues resource documents regarding safety and operations. Federal regulations establish weather guidelines for safe flying. The U.S. Department of

Transportation provides guidelines regarding standards of care. The Commission on Accreditation of Medical Transport Systems establishes voluntary accreditation standards, but air medical services associated with hospitals must meet hospital accreditation standards, typically those of the Joint Commission.

Safe Extrication from a Motor Vehicle (Car, Truck)

Scene management at the site of an accident that requires vehicle extrication incudes initial evaluation of any hazards at the site (360° evaluation), such as oncoming traffic, fallen wires, spilled fuel, and fire/explosion risk or presence. The scene must be secured (45° parking, police security, flares, and cones) and the EMT should don protective equipment as necessary and access the patient to provide life-saving care. The patient must be disentangled from the motor vehicle as much as can be done safely. The patient is prepared for extrication (such as by applying pressure to bleeding sites and placing a cervical collar), removed from the vehicle, and then prepared for ground or air transport and provided emergent treatment. For extrications in difficult terrain, assess the following:

- Terrain: Forests, desert, cliff, water, snow.
- Obstacles: Trees, rocks, light, unavailability of landing sites.
- Methods to be used: Helicopter extrication, overland carry, type of extrication.
- Alternative solutions: Abort; contact search and rescue.
- Safety issues: Review all safety concerns.

For **vehicle extrication,** the vehicle must be stabilized before the EMS personnel attempt to enter the vehicle or administer aid to the patient, especially if the vehicle may slide or is on its side and the personnel must access the vehicle from the top because the vehicle may shift and further endanger the patient as well as EMS personnel. EMS personnel can access the vehicle through a window (breaking it if necessary) or a door if one is operable (the patient may be able to assist in opening a window or door). EMS personnel should carry an airway (in case the patient requires ventilation), dressings (to apply pressure if the patient is bleeding), and a rigid cervical collar (to protect against spinal injury or further spinal damage) and should do rapid triage on access to the patient. Oxygen is usually not administered until after the patient is extracted because of the danger of fire, especially if the patient is saturated with fuel, and CPR is not done until the patient is in the supine position on a solid surface. If patients are apneic and pulseless, they must be removed as quickly as possible even with only manual protection of the spine being provided.

For **vehicle extrication**, once EMS personnel have gained access to the motor vehicle, they should unlock its doors if possible to allow others to more easily gain access. The EMS personnel should ensure that the engine is turned off, the parking brake is set, and the transmission is set to park. If possible, an emergency response person should disconnect the battery to decrease the risk of fire and explosion. If the patient can be removed, a short backboard should be applied before moving the patient. If the patient is wedged between the seat and the steering wheel, the seat may be slid back manually while rescuers support the patient. If the seat has become dislodged from the track, then the patient should be completely immobilized because this type of mechanical damage can result in severe physical injury. If the patient's legs are trapped, lifting the steering wheel away may also lift the dashboard and help to release the patient.

If a patient must be **cut from a vehicle** (such as when the vehicle is on its side and access must be through a U-shaped flap in the roof), he or she should be warned of the noise and should be covered with a safety blanket (heavy aluminized). In some accidents, **air bags** may not deploy, but movement of the patient or vehicle may cause them to deploy, resulting in danger to the patient and

EMS personnel. If the air bags have not deployed, then the battery cables should be disconnected or cut (negative side first) to prevent deployment and personnel should avoid being in front of the path of deployment. EMS personnel should check for side air bags as well as front. The air bags should be deactivated before the steering column is moved (keeping in mind that deactivation can take up to 30 minutes), and care should be taken to avoid cutting or drilling into an air bag.

Since the 1990s, vehicles have been equipped with **seat belt pretensioners** on three-point (shoulder harness) systems in the front and often also in the back. The purpose of seat belt pretensioners is to tighten any slack in the belts in an accident, pulling the person back into the seat and in the proper position for deployment of the air bag. Evidence of pretensioners is not always visible, although an accordion sleeve near the buckle end may be an indication. This sleeve compresses if the pretensioner fires. Although an undeployed pretensioner poses less threat to EMS personnel than an undeployed air bag, it can increase the risk of injury to the patient or EMS personnel, so the seat belt should be disconnected or cut immediately on access to the patient. If the patient was not wearing the seat belt on impact and the pretensioner fired, the seat belt will be tightly vertical along pillar B. If the seat belt pretensioner fired while being worn, it will be extended and will not be retractable.

Although large and heavy pieces of equipment, such as hydraulic rescue tools (including the Jaws of Life, cutters, spreaders, truck jacks, and rams), pneumatic tools, and come-along tools, are often used in vehicle extrication, a tool kit with **simple hand tools** should also be readily available. They may also be needed to access and safely remove a patient from a vehicle. Tools that may be needed for disassembly include adjustable wrenches, screwdrivers (flat and Phillips), flashlight, penlight, medical scissors, headlamp, pliers, bolt cutters, hammers, axes, crowbars, rescue knives (specially designed to cut through seat belts and clothing), and tin snips. Combination rescue tools are available that can be used for a variety of purposes, such as shutting off gas valves, prying open windows, and cutting through battery cables. Tool belt pouches are available to hold small tools that may be needed during an extrication.

Cribbing and chocking are used to raise a vehicle and prevent it from rolling, such as when a patient is caught beneath a vehicle. Cribbing consists of 2×4 blocks and wedges and 4×4 blocks and wedges that are used to create crib boxes to hold an air bag. Cribs are usually made of Douglas fir or southern yellow pine, which can hold 500 psi and crushes slowly. The cribbing is stacked with a 4-inch overhang (to allow for compression), and it should not exceed 48 inches in height. The crib box is put in place with the air bag on top. Chocks are large stepped wedges that are placed in front of or behind wheels to keep them from rolling when the air bag is inflated. As the air bag is slowly inflated, capture cribbing stacks are placed on both sides behind it to hold the vehicle when the air bag is deflated. Once the vehicle is elevated and secured, the air bag is deflated and the crib box is removed to allow room for extrication of the patient.

Some vehicles are powered by **alternative fuels**, such as compressed natural gas (CNG) or liquefied natural gas (LNG), so EMS personnel should look for CNG/LNG logos, often on the right rear or near the refueling port or the right rear of the cab (semitruck). A "natural gas vehicle" warning may be located near the bottom of the rear doors. CNG tanks may be located behind the cabs in semitractors, and some may have additional saddle tanks. The power should be turned off, and the 12-volt battery positive and negative cables should be cut. The emergency shut-off valve should be located and turned off, although each tank can also be turned off manually. Electric vehicles pose the risk of stranded energy. Batteries should always be considered energized with a potential for high-voltage injury. Damaged lithium ion batteries that are leaking or sparking are at risk for thermal runaway (fire). The car battery should be shut down immediately. If the battery is damaged, the vehicle must be relocated at least 50 feet from any combustible material.

Bus Extrication

Before accessing patients involved in a **bus crash,** the bus must be stabilized, especially if it is on its side or if it is upside down. If the engine is still running, a stop button is often located on the left side of the front panel. Access to the bus may be through the front door if possible. Access may also be through the front windshield (which can be removed through removal of the rubber locking strip that surrounds the window), side windows, the emergency exit door or window, the bathroom window, or an opening cut into the top of the vehicle. Removal of injured patients (usually on stretchers) from inside the vehicle often requires rapid triage and the assistance of multiple EMS personnel. If the vehicle remains upright but patients are completely or partially beneath the vehicle, they should be removed quickly because they may be crushed if the air suspension system deflates.

Aircraft Extrication

Communication is essential if EMS personnel are responding to an **aircraft crash site** because they need to know when the crash occurred, the type and size of the aircraft, the number of passengers and crew, reports of fire or explosion, and whether the aircraft is private, commercial, or military, as well as the status (fire, collapse) of any structure(s) that the aircraft may have impacted. For a small plane with the cabin still reasonably intact, extrication may be similar to a motor vehicle, but severe crashes in which the cabin is destroyed and large airplane crashes pose significantly different problems because passengers may have been thrown about inside or outside of the aircraft and seats and belongings and body parts may block access. Victims may lie in the roadway, so emergency vehicles must proceed with caution. Fire and explosions may be a severe risk, and rescuers may need to wait for fire suppression. Triage may begin outside of the aircraft while the aircraft (or the remains of the aircraft) is secured.

Extrication Considerations

Part of the stabilization of the scene is ensuring that it is secure. An outer perimeter is established to block public and media access, and an inner perimeter is established immediately about the scene of the rescue and the working crew. Three **control zones** are established as follows:

- Hot (coded red): This encompasses the inner perimeter and the crew as well as any area that is dangerous, such as an area contaminated by hazardous material or one in danger of a release of toxins.
- Warm (coded orange): Area for trained personnel in support of those in the hot zone. Decontamination of patients, crew, and equipment is carried out in this zone.
- Cold (coded yellow): This is the staging area and the command post (if necessary for the emergent situation). No members of the public or media should be allowed in the cold zone.

Zones are usually established by placement of police cars and fire-line tape.

The **path of least resistance** is an important concept to understand for rescues, especially if they involve fire and any products of combustion (smoke, heat, gas). Fire's path of least resistance is usually vertical and upward, although fire also spreads horizontally, especially if a vertical path is not available. It's for this reason that if there is a fire on the top floor of a building, the roof is breached to prevent horizontal spread. External factors, such as gusts of wind, can affect the path of least resistance. Water, on the other hand, also flows vertically, but downward and then horizontally if the downward flow is blocked. If the EMT is rescuing patients from a building, they will often be found near the path of least resistance, such as a near a door or window. Patients should also be transported according to the path of least resistance, that is, the route that is the easiest and safest.

Multistep Rescue Process

The **multistep rescue process** includes the following 10 steps:

1. Preparation: Training, readying equipment, and preparing for different types of rescues.
2. Response: Using protocols for dispatch; contacting others, such as utility companies, which may have the necessary knowledge or equipment.
3. Situation size-up: 360° site survey to identify hazards and determine the need for additional personnel or equipment. Determine if the situation is rescuer/equipment intensive.
4. Stabilization: Establishing perimeters and control zones, monitoring hazardous atmosphere, carrying out lockout/tagout of industrial equipment.
5. Access: Gaining access to the patient and providing emergent care.
6. Disentanglement: Freeing the patient.
7. Removal: Continuing critical and life support while assisting the patient to move or carrying the immobilized patient. Rapid extraction if his or her condition is life threatening.
8. Transport: Transporting by various means with decontamination done as needed.
9. Scene security: Police or others providing protection of the scene, crew, and patients.
10. Postevent analysis: Reviewing the procedures performed and the problems encountered.

Occupational Safety and Health Administration (OSHA)

The **Occupational Safety and Health Administration** (OSHA) is part of the U.S. Department of Labor, and it is charged with ensuring safe, healthful working conditions and setting and enforcing workplace standards. OSHA covers most employers in the private sector, but state and federal safety regulations also generally conform to OSHA standards. Employers must provide safety training, inform workers of chemical hazards, and provide required PPE. OSHA must be notified of a workplace-related death within 8 hours and a workplace-related injury that results in hospitalization, the loss of an eye, or amputation within 24 hours. Workers may file a complaint about workplace conditions with OSHA and request an inspection. OSHA's Whistleblower Protection Program prohibits retaliation by the employer. OSHA provides Hazardous Waste Operations and Emergency Response Standard (HAZWOPER) training courses (8-hour, 24-hour, 40-hour, and refresher) for first responders. OSHA has established regulations and guidelines that are industry specific. For example, OSHA has regulations regarding EMS. OSHA requires that hazardous material be color coded, with red indicating danger; yellow, caution; orange, warning; and fluorescent orange/orange-red, biological hazard.

Hazardous Materials and Exposure

Hazardous materials are any that may cause harm to humans or animals by themselves or through interaction with something else. Hazardous materials may be any of the following:

- Chemical: Include blister agents, blood agents, choking agents, nerve agents, asphyxiants, and irritants. These can enter the body through inhalation, absorption, ingestion, and injection.
- Radiological: Nuclear material and radioactive substances (alpha/beta particles).
- Physical/Biological: Infectious wastes, blood and other body fluids, and biotoxins.

Almost any material or substance can be classified as hazardous depending on various factors such as its location, amount, and interactions. Exposure occurs when a person/animal comes in contact with the hazardous material, and <u>contamination</u> is the residue resulting from exposure. <u>Absorption</u> is the method by which hazardous material enters the bloodstream. Exposure and contamination may result in an immediate response (blistering, itching, and pain) or a delayed response (nausea, vomiting, cancer, and lung disease).

The Environmental Protection Agency (EPA) classifies **hazardous wastes** according to the following characteristics:

- <u>Ignitable:</u> Liquids and nonliquids that can ignite and cause fires with flash points of <60°C/140°F.
- <u>Corrosive:</u> Based on pH (<2 or >12.5) or its ability to corrode steel.
- <u>Reactive:</u> Wastes that are unstable, may react with water, or that may result in toxic gases. They may also explode.
- <u>Toxic:</u> Heavy metal compounds that are harmful if ingested or absorbed.

Wastes may also be classified as listed wastes. These include wastes from manufacturing and industrial processes. Hazardous wastes are often produced in manufacturing, nuclear power plants (nuclear wastes), and healthcare facilities (needles and materials contaminated with body fluids). Nuclear wastes are classified as mixed waste because they contain a radioactive component as well as a hazardous component. Hazardous wastes can result in disease (such as from needle punctures), injury (from fire and explosions), and death (from toxic exposure and disease).

The purpose of **hazardous waste site characterization** is to identify hazards and select the appropriate PPE. The team leader is responsible for the assessment, but he or she may request assistance from outside experts, such as chemists. The three steps to hazardous waste site characterization include the following:

1. <u>Off-site characterization:</u> Gather information/data before personnel enter the site, including the location, a description of the activities, the duration of the event, terrain information (photographs, maps), habitation/population data, accessibility, paths of least resistance, and properties of any hazardous materials/substances. Conduct the needed interviews and review of records. Perimeter reconnaissance is done with observations, air sampling, and development of a preliminary site map.
2. <u>On-site survey:</u> Verify the information gathered from perimeter reconnaissance, survey the area and situation, note potential exposure to hazardous materials (dust, liquid, dead animals, gas) and safety hazards (obstacles, terrain, poisonous plants), and develop a site safety plan. The entry team should have at least four members: two to enter and two for outside support who can enter the site in an emergency.
3. <u>Ongoing monitoring:</u> Monitoring should be continuous.

Chemical Hazardous Waste Materials

Types of **chemical hazardous waste materials** include the following:

- Blister agents: Include sulfur mustard (mustard gas) and nitrogen mustard, which are both highly toxic. Exposure by inhalation, contact, or ingestion results in skin (erythema and blistering) and eye irritation and injury to the respiratory system as well as bone marrow suppression and gastrointestinal and neurological damage. The patient should be decontaminated within 1 to 2 minutes by flushing the eyes with water for up to 20 minutes and removing clothing and showering with soap (if available) and water for 20 minutes. Rescuers should use a self-contained breathing apparatus (SCBA), PPE (including eye protection), and chemical-protective gloves.
- Asphyxiants: Gas exposure (such as by butane, helium, and propane) lowers oxygen levels and results in suffocation. Patients require oxygen administration and may need CPR. This is especially a risk in confined spaces. Rescuers should use an SCBA.
- Blood agents: These include cyanide chloride, hydrogen cyanide, and arsine. Exposure by inhalation or ingestion. They prevent oxygen transfer from blood to cells. The patient may need oxygen and antidote. Rescuers should use an SCBA.
- Carcinogens: Agents such as asbestos, nickel compounds, and ionizing radiation that result in genetic mutation and cancer. There are various types of exposure. Patients must be removed from exposure. The rescuer must wear adequate PPE, and in some cases, he or she should use a mask or SCBA.
- Choking agents: Often, a chemical weapon is used (ammonia, chlorine) that is designed to inhibit breathing and incapacitate the person. Exposure is by inhalation, contact, or ingestion (rare). They may be corrosive to the skin and result in fluid in the lungs, leading to suffocation. Patients require supportive treatment and oxygen. Rescuers should use PPE and SCBA for most agents.
- Convulsants/Nerve agents: These include hydrazine and strychnine. Exposure may be by inhalation, contact, and ingestion. The severity of convulsions and nervous system impairment is dose related. Patients require supportive treatment. Rescuers need SCBA and protective suits (according to the exposure level of the agent).

Safety Data Sheets (SDSs)

Safety data sheets (SDSs), formerly known as material safety data sheets (MSDSs), explain how to handle caustic substances in the event of an accident or injury and provide pertinent information on the composition and toxic effects of chemicals in a lab. SDSs outline the proper storage of chemicals, procedures for the cleanup and dumping of caustic substances, procedures in the event of a chemical spill or injury, and the proper locations in the facility for cleanup. The SDS should also contain information indicating which substances may cause allergic effects or asthma from contact or inhalation. Emergency rescue services should obtain SDSs for common chemicals and products. Manufacturers and suppliers should have SDSs on file and can be contacted for copies. The OSHA/ Environmental Protection Agency (EPA) Occupational Chemical Database provides links for SDSs for some products. SDSs are available from various other sources, including the Toxicology Data Network (TOXNET) and poison control centers. There are also pathogen safety data sheets for biological hazards.

Multiple-Casualty Incidents Versus Mass-Casualty Incidents

Multiple-casualty incident	Mass-casualty incident
Involves more than one person, but different jurisdictions may quantify the total number of persons differently. Usually refers to an incident involving at least three patients. Usually involves only one jurisdiction and only one to three agencies (ambulance, fire department, and police). Requires triage, but generally only primary. Standards of care are maintained, and all patients not coded black (deceased) are transported for care.	Also involves more than one person, but may involve much larger numbers—dozens, hundreds, to thousands. Often involves multiple jurisdictions and agencies. Requires triage but may also involve separate waiting areas for color-coded individuals and secondary triage. Standards of care may be modified, and patients coded black (expectant) and not expected to live may be left in the field and/or receive delayed care if they are still living after the red- and yellow-coded individuals are transported.

Role of the Transportation Officer in a Mass-Casualty Incident

During a mass-casualty event, the **transportation officer** must maintain constant communication with hospitals and trauma centers, triage officers, police, ground ambulance services, and air medical transport services. The transportation officer controls the flow of patients for treatment and must determine where to route patients in order to prevent a backlog at the receiving facility and must coordinate incoming and outgoing ambulances in the transportation staging area. The transportation officer must obtain information about each facility's surge capacity and the number and types of patients the facility is prepared to care for. The transportation officer must also coordinate air medical transport flights and determine, with the triage officer, which patients to transport by air according to their severity of injuries, availability of treatment options, and appropriate levels of care. Speed of transportation and care is often critical in a mass-casualty incident because delays often result in increased death rates.

Role of Triage in a Mass-Casualty Incident Related to Terrorism or a Disaster

In a mass-casualty incident related to terrorism or a disaster, **rapid triage** and tagging must occur and patients must be sorted according to priority for transportation or field treatment. Because of the large numbers of casualties, triage should begin with the first patient encountered, proceeding from one to another. According to some plans, patients who are alive but expected to die are coded red, but this can result in overtriage, with too many red-coded individuals having to be transported and/or treated, resulting in patients dying during the wait. With other plans, patients expected to die are black-coded as "expectant" and left in the field or left aside until red- and yellow-coded individuals are transported and/or treated. If patients are undertriaged (such as patients who should be coded red being coded yellow instead) this can also result in increased deaths while other patients are waiting for transport and/or treatment.

Increasing Survival in Mass-Casualty Shooting and Improvised Explosive Device Incidents

Terrorist or other attacks that involve active shooters or improvised explosive devices (IEDs) often result in injuries similar to those encountered in combat situations in which the most common causes of death are extremity hemorrhage, tension pneumothorax, and airway obstruction. The **THREAT acronym** provides guidance for dealing with these situations in the following ways:

- Threat suppression: Use of police protection, ballistic vests, concealment, cover, and situational awareness. One concern is that most of the protective gear available to emergency medical personnel is for ballistics rather than explosive devices.
- Hemorrhage control: Use of tourniquets (military style) and hemostatic dressings (QuikClot) to control bleeding.
- Rapid extrication to safety: Move patients and personnel out of the danger zone to prevent further injuries.
- Assessment by medical providers: Includes provision of a nasopharyngeal airway or upright seating and leaning forward for airway compromise and spinal precautions.
- Transport to definitive care: Medical treatment should continue during transport.

Safety Issues Associated with Active Shooters and Terrorist Bomb Attacks

With **active shooters,** standard protocol has been for emergency response services to wait until the police have removed the threat and secured the area before moving in to care for victims; however, this delay in treatment may result in death, so some authorities are now recommending that emergency response personnel enter the scene with police while wearing appropriate protective equipment, although this does pose some risk, especially with additional shooters or a secondary attack. With a **terrorist bombing** and improvised explosive devices (IEDs), situational awareness is critical because multiple explosive devices (some undetonated) may be at the scene. IEDs may be inside backpacks, suitcases, and packages left unattended, but in emergency situations, innocent people often drop backpacks and packages and run away. Additionally, attackers wearing suicide vests or belts may mix in with other victims or people escaping the blast area.

Bomb Threat Standoff Recommendations

Threat	Explosive capacity (lb)	Mandatory evacuation distance (ft)	Preferred evacuation distance (ft)	Shelter-in-place zone (ft)
Pipe bomb	5	70	1200+	71–1199
Suicide bomber	20	110	1700+	111–1699
Suitcase /Briefcase	50	150	1850+	151–1849
Automobile	500	320	1900+	321–1899
SUV/Van	1000	400	2400+	401–2399
Small truck	4000	640	3800+	641–3799
Container truck	10,000	860	5100+	861–5099
Semitrailer	60,000	1570	9300+	1571–9299

Source: U.S. Department of Homeland Security.

B-NICE Hazardous Material (Hazmat) Incidents Associated with Terrorist Attacks

Category	Response
B—Biological (bacteria, viruses, fungi, toxins)	Inhalation type—evacuate for 80 feet, shut down air-handling systems, wear appropriate PPE and SCBA, and avoid contamination. Visible agent—decontaminate with soap and water. Symptoms may vary but are usually delayed.
N—Nuclear/ Radiological	Inhalation type (most common)—Isolate/Secure the area, avoid smoke/fumes, stay upwind, and use PPE and SCBA. Isolate victims and decontaminate as appropriate. Symptoms are usually delayed.
I—Incendiary	Be on alert for multiple devices and sabotaged fire suppression equipment. Symptoms include burns, pain, and trauma.
C—Chemical	Isolate/Secure the area, decontaminate victims with soap and water, and be on alert for chemical dispersal devices. Approach toward uphill and upwind. Isolate symptomatic patients from others. Symptoms vary but may include burns, blistering, vomiting, breathing difficulty, and neurological damage.
E—Explosives	Be alert for secondary devices, undetonated devices, and secondary hazards (unstable buildings and debris). Remove victims from the area, secure the perimeter, and stage away from the incident area. Decontaminate as necessary. Symptoms include burns, amputations, cuts, and penetrating and blunt trauma.

"All-Hazards" Safety Approach to Mass-Casualty Incidents

The **"all-hazards" safety approach** to mass-casualty incidents aims to provide plans that can be used to deal with all types of hazards (natural disasters, terrorist attacks, and mass-casualty incidents) as well as encompassing the four components of emergency management: mitigation, preparedness, response, and recovery. Organizations in an area coordinate to develop joint action plans that can be activated in response to incidents, with the chain of command clearly outlined. This approach lowers costs to individual organizations and provides for faster and more effective response. However, although the basic structure may be the same for responding to all hazards, there are inevitable differences between (for example) a terrorist attack with active shooters and a natural disaster, such as a hurricane, which can be anticipated and mitigated to some degree. For this reason, modifying existing incident action plans to meet the needs of a situation is essential.

Treating Terrorists and Criminals

In mass-casualty incidents, **terrorists and criminals** involved in the incident may be injured and require treatment, and EMS personnel may feel conflicted about providing treatment when others have been injured or killed, but it's important to provide treatment to terrorists and criminals the same as any other individuals because (1) they are in need of help and (2) their survival may be critical to identifying coconspirators and to providing reasons for the attack. However, these individuals may pose risks to emergency medical personnel, so they should be examined while under police guard. The individual's hands should be examined first to check for weapons and detonators and secured (with handcuffs, if possible). Clothes should be examined and removed very carefully in case the person is wearing a suicide device of some type. Emergency medical personnel should also be aware that the individual may be feigning injury or unconsciousness.

EMT Practice Test

Questions 1 to 3 pertain to the following scenario:

> You and your partner are called to the home of a 75-year-old man complaining of severe pain in the chest and nausea. As the patient is being assessed, he suddenly loses consciousness.

1. The first step in treating a patient with severe chest pain is:
   a. obtain a patient history.
   b. administer oxygen.
   c. perform a physical exam.
   d. obtain baseline vital signs.

2. The first step in treating a patient who loses consciousness is to:
   a. obtain a pulse.
   b. assess breathing.
   c. attach an automated external defibrillator.
   d. open the airway.

3. The best way to decrease oxygen demand in the case of cardiac compromise is to:
   a. transport the patient immediately, flashing lights and using siren.
   b. reassure the patient.
   c. travel at high speed but without the siren.
   d. give the patient nitroglycerin.

Questions 4 to 6 pertain to the following scenario:

> You receive a call from the mother of a 3-year-old girl. The mother believes her daughter has "swallowed something." When you arrive, the child does not acknowledge your presence. She has a high fever and a generalized rash.

4. Proper care for a small child with possible airway obstruction consists of:
   a. performing a finger sweep.
   b. relieving mild airway obstruction.
   c. avoiding agitation of the child and providing transport.
   d. applying back blows and abdominal thrusts.

5. When a young child does not acknowledge the presence of a stranger in his or her environment, this is indicative of:
   a. altered mental state.
   b. allergic reaction.
   c. sleep.
   d. age-appropriate behavior.

6. A child with inattentive behavior, high fever, and generalized rash should be monitored for:

    a. dehydration.
    b. projectile vomiting.
    c. cardiac failure.
    d. seizures.

7. In which of the following patients is rapid trauma assessment most urgently needed?

    a. A 90-year-old woman with pain in the right upper quadrant.
    b. A conscious 50-year-old man who fell from the roof of his home and landed on his left arm.
    c. A conscious 25-year-old store clerk who was stabbed in the abdomen during an attempted robbery.
    d. An 8-year-old boy complaining of pain in the right lower quadrant of the abdomen.

8. You receive a call from a young woman whose car has been struck in a shopping mall parking lot. She is concerned about the elderly man who backed into her car. On arrival at the scene, you find a conscious 88-year-old man who appears to be having an acute ischemic stroke. The most appropriate course of action would be to:

    a. perform a physical exam.
    b. administer oxygen and obtain a patient history.
    c. monitor blood pressure.
    d. administer oxygen and provide transport to the hospital for fibrinolytic therapy.

Questions 9 and 10 refer to the following scenario:

> The husband of a pregnant 21-year-old woman calls for assistance, fearing that his wife is about to deliver "any minute." On arrival, delivery does not appear to be imminent; however, during transport, crowning occurs.

9. The most appropriate course of action is to:

    a. check for the presence of the amniotic sac.
    b. reassure the mother and wait for arrival at the hospital.
    c. apply gentle pressure to the infant's head.
    d. gently slide the infant back into the birth canal.

10. On delivery, the infant is not breathing adequately and the umbilical cord is pulsating. You should immediately:

    a. pull on the umbilical cord.
    b. leave the umbilical cord attached until arrival at the hospital.
    c. clamp and cut the umbilical cord.
    d. clamp the umbilical cord and await arrival at the hospital.

Questions 11 to 13 pertain to the following scenario:

The manager of a fast-food restaurant calls to report that an elderly woman is choking. On arrival, you find an 80-year-old woman in a wheelchair in obvious respiratory distress. On breathing assessment, you observe that the patient's dentures are loose and ill-fitting. She then begins to make gurgling sounds.

11. The first step in evaluating the airway of an elderly person is to:

   a. extend the head and flex the neck.
   b. thrust the jaw forward to pull the tongue out of the airway.
   c. find a radial pulse.
   d. suction for 30 seconds.

12. While evaluating the airway, you notice there may be some difficulty in ventilating the patient. You should proceed by:

   a. removing the patient's dentures.
   b. suctioning for 30 seconds.
   c. initiating the gag reflex.
   d. offering high-concentration oxygen.

13. The presence of gurgling sounds in this patient indicates that:

   a. the patient is in cardiac arrest.
   b. the patient is in an altered mental state.
   c. the patient requires suctioning.
   d. the patient is having an acute ischemic attack.

14. You arrive at the home of a 75-year-old woman who has had a fall. In addition to assessing potential injuries, you should:

   a. assess mental status.
   b. oxygenate the patient.
   c. assess potential causes of the fall.
   d. assess circulation.

15. Which of the following drugs are most often carried on an ambulance?

   a. Nitroglycerin
   b. Epinephrine
   c. Inhalers
   d. Oral glucose

16. Which of the following drugs can an EMT-B assist a patient in taking?

   a. Nitroglycerin
   b. Amitriptyline
   c. Verapamil
   d. Nifedipine

Questions 17 to 19 pertain to the following scenario:

> You are called to the scene of a traffic accident involving a mother and her 2-year-old son. On arrival, both mother and child are bleeding from the head. The mother is conscious and alert and informs you that while she has sustained "just a scratch," her son is "seriously hurt." The boy has a laceration on the top of his head. On examination, he exhibits signs of hypoperfusion.

17. One of the most common causes of hypoperfusion in infants and children is:

    a. heart failure.
    b. blood loss.
    c. a stressful event.
    d. lack of oxygen.

18. Which of the following is a sign of hypoperfusion in children?

    a. Crying.
    b. Rapid pulse.
    c. Rapid respiratory rate.
    d. Increased urinary output.

19. The best course of care for this child is to:

    a. wait for signs of decompensated shock.
    b. perform airway clearance.
    c. monitor blood pressure.
    d. keep the child warm.

20. The most likely cause of cardiac arrest in a child is:

    a. respiratory failure.
    b. hypothermia.
    c. mitral valve prolapse.
    d. asthma attack.

Questions 21 to 23 pertain to the following scenario:

> The morning after a snow storm, the ski patrol discover the wreckage of an automobile on the road to a ski lodge. A 70-year-old man is trapped inside. He is disoriented but conscious and has suffered a broken hip. He exhibits severe muscular rigidity and has no memory of the events before or after the accident. The patient's wife had reported the man missing the previous night after he became intoxicated and was ejected from a local bar.

21. In addition to a broken hip, this patient is suffering from:

    a. hypoperfusion.
    b. inadequate circulation.
    c. hypothermia.
    d. psychiatric disorder.

- 144 -

22. To prevent heat loss in an injured patient, you should:

   a. perform active rewarming techniques.
   b. massage the extremities.
   c. administer a stimulant.
   d. use blankets to provide a barrier to the outside.

23. Body heat loss is often associated with:

   a. alcohol intoxication.
   b. head trauma.
   c. cardiac events.
   d. altered mental status.

24. The signs and symptoms of carbon monoxide poisoning most closely resemble those of:

   a. smoke inhalation.
   b. flu.
   c. food poisoning.
   d. drug overdose.

25. You receive an urgent call from the mother of a 15-year-old-boy who has accidentally splashed disinfectant in his eye while performing his weekly chore of cleaning the bathroom. The best way to treat the boy is to:

   a. irrigate the eye with clean water for 20 minutes if an alkali or 10 minutes if an acid.
   b. irrigate the eye with diluted vinegar.
   c. irrigate the eye with baking soda and water.
   d. transport the patient to the hospital immediately.

Questions 26 to 28 pertain to the following scenario:

   You receive a call from a distraught 18-year-old girl. Her parents are away for the weekend and she is having an illicit party during which alcohol and other substances have been consumed. Her 16-year-old brother has slipped and hit his head on the coffee table. The boy has a contusion on the side of his head. He is conscious but has slurred speech and appears confused. He denies having consumed any alcohol or drugs.

26. In addition to alcohol intoxication, slurred speech and confusion may be signs of:

   a. altered mental state.
   b. head injury.
   c. seizure.
   d. drug overdose.

27. The best course of action in this case would be to:

   a. transport the patient to the hospital.
   b. call the police.
   c. ask the patient again if he has been using drugs.
   d. call the parents.

28. The patient suddenly becomes violent and begins to throw objects around the room. Your reaction should be to:

    a. reassure the patient.
    b. restrain the patient.
    c. go to a safe place and call the police.
    d. call the parents.

29. Which of the following indicates correct placement of an endotracheal tube?

    a. Presence of breath sounds only in the epigastrium
    b. Presence of breath sounds on the right apex
    c. Presence of breath sounds on the left apex
    d. Presence of breath sounds on both the right and left

30. Which of the following does **not** affect the accuracy of an oximeter reading?

    a. Cigarette smoking
    b. Hypothermia
    c. Carbon monoxide poisoning
    d. Fever

Questions 31 to 33 pertain to the following scenario:

> The wife of a 65-year-old man calls, fearing that her husband is "having a heart attack." When you arrive, the man is conscious, but sweating profusely and complaining of chest pain. He tells you the pain developed while he was mowing the lawn. When asked if he is taking any medications, he says he has been on nitroglycerin, and that although he took the "maximum dose," it did not alleviate the chest pain. After taking his vital signs, you observe that his pulse is 130 beats per minute and blood pressure is 200/100. The patient gives you permission to transport him to the hospital.

31. According to SAMPLE, the information you should always obtain from patient includes:

    a. medication history.
    b. insurance information.
    c. physician's name.
    d. emergency contact information.

32. Profuse sweating in a patient is an example of a

    a. symptom.
    b. sign.
    c. drug overdose.
    d. medication side effect.

33. Nitroglycerin is often prescribed for patients with:

    a. congestive heart failure.
    b. clogged arteries.
    c. angina pectoris.
    d. arrhythmia.

34. Compared with adults, infants and children have:

    a. slower pulse.
    b. higher blood pressure.
    c. slower respiratory rate.
    d. lower blood pressure.

35. You are called to the home of a 75-year-old woman who has stopped breathing. Her husband requests that you do not resuscitate the patient because she has terminal cancer. Your procedure should include:

    a. not resuscitate the patient as her husband requests.
    b. contact medical direction.
    c. try to resuscitate the patient.
    d. transport the patient to the hospital.

36. While off duty, you observe a severe car accident, with one of the vehicles overturned. Your procedure should include:

    a. provide care to the victims, then leave the scene.
    b. provide care and wait for additional help to arrive.
    c. call 911 and leave the scene.
    d. begin care, call for additional help, then leave the scene.

37. Which of the following is **not** useful in assessing an unresponsive adult patient with head trauma?

    a. Mental status
    b. Airway obstruction
    c. Capillary refill
    d. Skin color

38. A dangerous pulse rate for an adult in an emergency situation would be:

    a. above 100 beats per minute.
    b. below 50 beats per minute.
    c. 60 beats per minute.
    d. 90 beats per minute.

39. A pulse rate of 120 beats per minute in a 3-year-old child is

    a. not a cause for concern.
    b. indicative of imminent cardiac arrest.
    c. indicative of accidental drug overdose.
    d. indicative of shock.

40. You have difficulty in finding the carotid pulse of an injured 5-year-old girl. You should:

    a. use your thumb.
    b. apply more pressure.
    c. assess the carotid pulse on the other side.
    d. assess the carotid pulse on both sides.

Questions 41 to 43 pertain to the following scenario:

> You are called to the scene of a traffic accident involving a 40-year-old woman. The patient is conscious but reports that her airbag deflated and she was thrown against the steering wheel. You notice a large cut on her forehead and bruising on her neck.

41. Because of her injuries, this patient is at risk of :
    a. shock.
    b. cervical spine injury.
    c. subdural hematoma.
    d. internal bleeding.

42. The first step in treating this patient is to:
    a. manually stabilize the head and neck.
    b. apply a soft collar.
    c. apply a rigid collar.
    d. secure the patient to a backboard.

43. Before you transport this patient to the hospital, you should:
    a. apply a soft collar.
    b. apply a rigid collar.
    c. palpate the back of the neck.
    d. tilt the head back.

44. A detailed physical examination is most often performed on:
    a. an accident victim with a broken leg.
    b. an elderly patient with a heart condition.
    c. an accident victim with head trauma.
    d. a child with airway obstruction.

45. In the case of a patient with chronic bronchitis in respiratory distress, the preferred course of action is to:
    a. withhold oxygen.
    b. provide artificial ventilation.
    c. place the patient in a supine position.
    d. administer oxygen.

Questions 46 to 48 pertain to the following scenario:

> You receive a call from the wife of a 66-year-old man with COPD. The man has been having difficulty breathing. When you arrive, he is making gurgling sounds and cannot speak. He appears disoriented and his skin is flushed.

46. Gurgling sounds in a patient with breathing difficulty are usually a sign of:
    a. open airway.
    b. obstruction.
    c. fluid in throat.
    d. stridor.

47. The typical position for COPD patients with breathing difficulty is:

    a. sitting with feet dangling.
    b. tripod position.
    c. lying down.
    d. hunching over.

48. Altered mental status in a patient who has difficulty breathing is usually a sign of:

    a. COPD.
    b. airway obstruction.
    c. lack of oxygen.
    d. cyanosis.

Questions 49 to 51 pertain to the following scenario:

> A 38-year-old woman falls through the ice while skating on a frozen pond with her 6-year-old daughter. While the child went to get help, her mother had been trapped waist-deep in the freezing water for several hours. After rescue, the woman reports that her toes are freezing. On assessment, her toes appear grayish-blue in color and feel frozen to the touch.

49. The first step in caring for this patient would be to:

    a. squeeze the toes to increase circulation.
    b. perform active rewarming.
    c. massage the toes to increase circulation.
    d. administer high-concentration oxygen.

50. Transport to the hospital has been severely delayed due to icy road conditions. A rescue worker offers the patient a drink of an alcoholic beverage from a flask to keep her warm. The next step in treating this patient should be to:

    a. continue to massage the frozen area.
    b. begin active rewarming.
    c. heat a container of water and immerse the patient's feet until they touch the bottom.
    d. keep the frozen area covered and allow the patient to sip the alcoholic beverage.

51. In the process of active rewarming, you should:

    a. put pressure on the affected area to rapidly increase circulation.
    b. allow the patient to walk on the affected area to increase circulation.
    c. keep the affected area immersed until the patient feels pain.
    d. keep the affected area wrapped in blankets until transport is available.

52. In rescuing a near-drowning victim, you should:

    a. perform chest compression.
    b. attempt rescue breathing while the victim is still in the water.
    c. remove the victim from the water before initiating care.
    d. immobilize the victim, then remove the victim from the water.

53. Emergency care for a snakebite includes:

    a. cleaning the bite with soap and water.
    b. placing ice on the bite.
    c. sucking the venom from the bite.
    d. capturing the snake.

54. Typical signs and symptoms in a heat emergency patient with hot and dry or moist skin include:

    a. heavy perspiration.
    b. little or no perspiration.
    c. muscle cramps.
    d. weak pulse.

55. Typical signs and symptoms in a heat emergency patient with normal or cool moist, pale skin include:

    a. rapid pulse.
    b. seizures.
    c. little or no perspiration.
    d. muscle cramps.

56. An example of a medical condition that can mimic a psychiatric condition is:

    a. heart attack.
    b. diabetes.
    c. asthma.
    d. allergic reaction.

57. Proper treatment of a hostile or aggressive patient includes:

    a. restraining the patient.
    b. encouraging the patient to accept emergency care.
    c. calling a physician.
    d. watching for sudden changes in behavior.

58. Proper restraint of a violent patient includes:

    a. Handcuffs.
    b. Plastic restraints.
    c. Leather cuffs.
    d. "Hog-tying."

59. Proper care for a child with epiglottitis should include:

    a. taking the child's temperature.
    b. putting the child in a supine position.
    c. inserting an oral airway.
    d. transporting the child to the hospital.

60. In treating an infant or child with fever, you should:

    a. apply rubbing alcohol to reduce the patient's temperature.
    b. transport the patient to the hospital.
    c. submerge the child in cold water.
    d. apply towels soaked in cold water.

Questions 61 to 63 pertain to the following scenario:

The mother of a 4-year-old boy calls you because her son is "unning a high fever. The boy has been vomiting and has diarrhea. His temperature is 103ºF.

61. The best line of treatment for a child with diarrhea and vomiting is to

    a. allow the child to sip some water or chipped ice.
    b. maintain an open airway and administer oxygen.
    c. insert an oropharyngeal airway.
    d. administer an antidiarrheal.

62. To first step in assessing a child with fever should be to:

    a. obtain an oral temperature.
    b. obtain a rectal temperature.
    c. determine the child's temperature using a skin thermometer.
    d. cover the child with towels soaked in tepid water.

63. On transport to the hospital, the child suddenly has a seizure. You should immediately:

    a. provide oxygen.
    b. insert an oropharyngeal airway.
    c. insert a bite stick.
    d. keep the child covered and wait until arrival at the hospital.

64. Signs of iron poisoning in a child include:

    a. hyperventilation.
    b. drowsiness.
    c. irritability.
    d. bloody vomiting.

65. In treating a child with meningitis, an EMT-B should always:

    a. assess for shock.
    b. call medical direction.
    c. wear a surgical mask.
    d. obtain a relative skin temperature.

66. Which of the following statements regarding use of the ambulance siren is FALSE?

    a. Use the siren when close to alert the driver of a vehicle ahead.
    b. Continuous use of a siren can increase an operator's driving speed.
    c. Use of a siren can make motorists less inclined to give the right of way.
    d. Use of a siren can worsen the condition of a patient.

67. En route to a call, an emergency vehicle is **NOT** allowed to:

    a. pass in a no-passing zone.
    b. exceed the speed limit.
    c. pass a school bus with red lights blinking.
    d. pass through a stop sign.

68. Which of the following statements regarding use of visual warning devices in an emergency vehicle is FALSE?

   a. Headlights should be kept on both day and night.
   b. Four-way flashers can be used as emergency lights.
   c. Alternating flashing headlights should only be used if attached to secondary head lamps.
   d. Lights should blink in tandem rather than in an alternating pattern.

69. Which of the following steps should be taken when transporting a patient to the hospital?

   a. More time should be spent packaging a highly traumatized patient.
   b. Sheets and blankets should be kept as loose as possible.
   c. Trauma patients should be secured to a spine board or other carrying device.
   d. A highly traumatized patient should not be moved until emergency treatment is completed.

70. Vital signs should be assessed:

   a. every 15 minutes in an unstable patient.
   b. every 5 minutes in an unstable patient.
   c. every 10 minutes in a stable patient.
   d. every 10 minutes in an unstable patient.

71. When transferring a patient without serious injury to the emergency department, you should:

   a. keep the patient in the ambulance until the operator decides where he or she should be taken.
   b. bring the patient directly into the emergency room, then leave the scene.
   c. place the patient in a hospital bed, then leave the scene.
   d. submit a prehospital care report, then leave the scene.

72. Which of the following statements regarding stabilization of a collision vehicle is TRUE?

   a. A vehicle upright on four wheels should be considered stable.
   b. The tires on an upright vehicle should be deflated.
   c. To stabilize a vehicle that has fallen on its side, kneel down to place cribbing.
   d. Stabilization is required in a vehicle with a crushed roof.

73. In the care of a patient with hazardous materials injuries, you should:

   a. make sure the patient has been decontaminated.
   b. transport the patient immediately.
   c. begin care only after the patient has been moved to a safe zone.
   d. wait for arrival of the hazardous materials (hazmat) team before treating the patient.

74. In initial triage, a patient in cardiac arrest is considered Priority 1 in the following situation:

   a. under all circumstances.
   b. in cases of severe hypothermia.
   c. in cases of cold water drowning.
   d. when ample resources are available.

75. In the case of a multiple-casualty incident, patients should be transported:

   a. immediately.
   b. only under the direction of a transportation officer.
   c. within 30 minutes of notification.
   d. under direction of radio dispatch.

76. A child's airway differs from that of an adult because:

    a. the tongue is smaller.
    b. the chest wall is more rigid.
    c. the tongue is larger.
    d. the trachea is wider.

77. Which sign of inadequate breathing is more often found in children than adults?

    a. seesaw breathing.
    b. cyanosis.
    c. diminished breath sounds.
    d. inability to speak.

78. Which of the following is **NOT** a complication of orotracheal intubation?

    a. Hypoxia
    b. Soft-tissue trauma
    c. Increased heart rate
    d. Decreased heart rate

79. What is the problem in the case of an infiltrated IV?

    a. the IV fluid flows into surrounding tissue.
    b. the IV flow rate is too fast.
    c. tubing is caught under the backboard.
    d. tubing has pulled out of the catheter.

80. A potentially serious sign or symptom associated with an acute stress reaction is:

    a. difficulty sleeping.
    b. nausea.
    c. loss of appetite.
    d. uncontrollable crying.

Questions 81 to 83 pertain to the following scenario:

> You are called to the scene of a car accident involving a 30-year-old woman and her 3-year-old son. The brakes on the car failed, causing the woman to hit a tree. Both the mother and her son have lost consciousness.

81. The first step in assessing the mother should be:

    a. perform CPR.
    b. determine responsiveness.
    c. open the airway.
    d. resuscitate for 1 minute, then activate EMS.

82. The first step in assessing the child should be:

    a. resuscitate for 1 minute, then activate EMS.
    b. open the airway.
    c. activate EMS.
    d. take a pulse.

- 153 -

83. To assess circulation in the child, you should:

    a. feel for the brachial artery.
    b. feel for the carotid artery.
    c. perform chest compression.
    d. perform CPR.

84. If an adult patient has stopped breathing but has a pulse, you should:

    a. perform chest compression.
    b. begin CPR.
    c. provide rescue breathing.
    d. open the airway.

85. To open the airway of an unconscious patient with a possible spinal injury:

    a. perform the head-tilt maneuver.
    b. perform the chin-lift maneuver.
    c. rotate the patient's head.
    d. perform the jaw-thrust maneuver.

86. In the case of a patient with gastric distention and vomiting, you should:

    a. turn the patient's head.
    b. roll the patient onto his side.
    c. place the patient in a supine position.
    d. perform rescue breathing.

87. The correct position for releasing chest compression should be to:

    a. place your hands on the patient's sternum and move from the hips.
    b. lift your hands away from the sternum.
    c. bend your elbows and lift your hands from the sternum.
    d. keep your knees and elbows bent.

88. Muscles connect to bones via which of the following:

    a. ligaments.
    b. nerves.
    c. myofibril.
    d. tendons.

89. In treating a laceration, you should:

    a. gently probe the edges of the laceration to see the extent of the wound.
    b. apply butterfly bandages and leave the patient in the emergency department.
    c. check the patient's pulse.
    d. bandage the laceration immediately.

90. In caring for a patient with a puncture wound from an impaled object, you should:

    a. remove the object.
    b. put pressure on the object.
    c. bandage the wounded area.
    d. stabilize the object.

91. The best way to save an avulsed body part is to:

    a. put the part in dry ice.
    b. immerse the part in ice water.
    c. wrap the part in a dry sterile dressing.
    d. immerse the part in saline.

92. Which of the following statements regarding abdominal bullet wounds is **TRUE**?

    a. An abdominal gunshot wound without an exit wound can be dangerous.
    b. Internal abdominal injury from a bullet wound can be easily detected.
    c. Only the area directly underneath an entrance wound may be seriously injured.
    d. Only the area directly underneath an exit wound may be seriously injured.

93. Which of the following statements regarding burns is **FALSE**?

    a. Chemical burns can burn continuously for days.
    b. Alkaline chemicals can enter the bloodstream via burns.
    c. The age of the patient should be considered when assessing burns.
    d. An electrical burn is usually not serious.

94. According to the rule of nines, which of the following is **TRUE?**

    a. an infant's head involves the same amount of body surface as an adult's.
    b. an infant's head accounts for 18% of body surface.
    c. each lower limb in an adult accounts for 13.5% of body surface.
    d. an adult's head accounts for 18% of body surface.

95. Which of the following types of burns can be treated by flushing with water?

    a. carbolic acid
    b. dry lime
    c. hydrofluoric acid
    d. electrical burns

96. Chemical burns to the eyes should be treated by:

    a. flushing with vinegar or baking soda.
    b. covering the eye with a moistened pad.
    c. flooding the eye with water for at least 20 minutes.
    d. covering the eye and transporting the patient.

97. In bandaging an open wound, you should take care to:

    a. cover the fingers and toes.
    b. leave the fingers and toes exposed.
    c. remove blood-soaked dressings.
    d. tightly bandage the wound.

Questions 98 to 100 pertain to the following scenario:

> You are called to the scene of a traffic accident involving a sport utility vehicle (SUV) and a city bus. The elderly driver of the SUV had suffered a heart attack behind the wheel and crashed into the bus. Of the 15 passengers on the bus, 5 have multiple bone injuries, 2 severe head trauma and bleeding, 2 difficulty breathing, 2 back

- 155 -

injuries, and 4 musculoskeletal or soft-tissue injuries. The bus driver has a probable spinal cord injury.

98. In initial triage, the 2 patients with breathing difficulties should be classified as:

    a. priority 2.
    b. priority 1.
    c. priority 4.
    d. priority 3.

99. The elderly driver of the SUV has gone into cardiac arrest. This patient should be classified as:

    a. priority 1.
    b. priority 4.
    c. priority 2.
    d. priority 3.

100. The bus driver should be classified as:

    a. priority 1.
    b. priority 4.
    c. priority 2.
    d. priority 3.

101. Which of the following is the correct sequence of connective function?

    a. Muscle-ligament-bone
    b. Bone-muscle-ligament
    c. Muscle-tendon-bone
    d. Muscle-bone-tendon

Questions 102 to 104 pertain to the following scenario:

> During an ice storm, the car of a 25-year-old man skids off the road and crashes into the side of a grocery store. His right arm is bleeding profusely, with the end of the bone protruding through the skin. The patient also reports severe pain in his right femur.

102. The first step in treating this patient is to:

    a. push the protruding bone back into place.
    b. assess for life-threatening injury.
    c. align the bone in a neutral position.
    d. transport to the hospital immediately.

103. The proper care for this patient's protruding bone is to:

    a. realign the injury and splint.
    b. push the bone back into place.
    c. immobilize the patient on a long spine board.
    d. splint the injury in the position in which it was found.

104. The best method of treatment for the patient's injured femur is to:

    a. use a rigid splint.
    b. use a formable splint.
    c. use a traction splint.
    d. immobilize the patient on a long spine board.

105. To treat an open abdominal injury, you should:

    a. apply an occlusive dressing using aluminum foil.
    b. replace any eviscerated or exposed organs.
    c. give the patient sips of water.
    d. apply a sterile saline dressing.

106. Which of the following statements regarding shoulder girdle injuries is **TRUE**?

    a. A dislocated shoulder can sometimes go back into place.
    b. Use a rigid splint for shoulder injuries.
    c. Always attempt to straighten out a dislocated shoulder.
    d. If spinal injury is suspected, tie a sling around the patient's neck.

107. A hip fracture is a fracture of the:

    a. pelvis.
    b. proximal femur.
    c. pubic bone.
    d. humerus bone.

108. In treating an ankle or foot injury, you should:

    a. apply manual traction.
    b. apply an ice pack directly to the skin.
    c. change the position of the ankle.
    d. tie a pillow to the ankle and foot.

109. Use of the PASG is indicated in cases of:

    a. cardiogenic shock.
    b. shock in the presence of a chest wound.
    c. pelvic injury.
    d. congestive heart failure.

110. A blood glucose meter reading of 145 indicates:

    a. hypoglycemia.
    b. hyperglycemia.
    c. diabetes.
    d. normal blood sugar level.

111. Which of the following statements is **FALSE**?

    a. A diabetic adult is at higher risk of a medical emergency than a diabetic child.
    b. Altered mental status may be caused by diabetes.
    c. Meningitis may cause altered mental status.
    d. Altered mental status may be associated with alcohol use.

112. According to the Ryan White act, if an EMT is possibly exposed to a bloodborne disease, which procedure should be followed:

a. A hospital is required to test the patient for bloodborne diseases if requested.
b. A hospital is required to review the patient's medical records for evidence of bloodborne disease.
c. A hospital is required to test the patient if requested by a designated officer.
d. The patient must be tested for disease within 48 hours.

113. Which of the following statements regarding consent is **FALSE**?

a. Care may be given to a child without parental consent.
b. Expressed consent must be given by all patients before treatment is given.
c. In the case of an unconscious patient, consent may be assumed.
d. A mentally impaired patient has the right to refuse treatment.

114. According to patient confidentiality requirements:

a. patient information can be disclosed if the patient grants verbal permission.
b. patient information cannot be shared with other healthcare personnel.
c. patient information can only be disclosed if the patient signs a written release.
d. patient information can be disclosed while calling medical direction.

115. A supine patient is positioned:

a. on the back.
b. on the abdomen.
c. on one side.
d. seated with legs straight out.

116. In the Trendelenburg position, the patient is in which state:

a. Lying on one side.
b. Lying on the abdomen.
c. Lying with the head lower than the feet.
d. Leaning back in a semi-seated position.

117. A fractured rib may cause:

a. shock.
b. cyanosis.
c. altered mental status.
d. inadequate breathing.

118. The preferred method for moving a patient down a set of stairs is to:

a. carry the patient on your back.
b. use a stair chair.
c. carry the patient on a stretcher.
d. lean forward from your hips.

119. Which of the following may be used to move a patient with suspected spinal injury?

a. Urgent moves
b. Extremity lift
c. Direct carry
d. Draw-sheet method

120. Which statement regarding the danger zone of an accident scene is **FALSE**?

    a. The danger zone extends at least 50 feet in all directions.
    b. Park the ambulance inside the danger zone to better assist victims.
    c. Park the ambulance away from the poles on which downed wires are attached.
    d. The size of the danger zone depends on the nature and severity of the accident.

121. As a BSI precaution, you should:

    a. determine the mechanism of injury.
    b. assess the crime scene.
    c. wear a protective mask.
    d. assess mental status.

122. A "fender-bender" occurs between two cars in a parking lot. Both drivers claim they are unhurt, although the male driver was thrown against the steering wheel on impact. The best course of action would be to:

    a. assume both drivers have sustained no injuries.
    b. identify the mechanism of injury and treat accordingly.
    c. treat only the driver who was thrown against the wheel.
    d. report the accident and leave the scene.

123. Which of the following does **NOT** indicate a life-threatening condition?

    a. inadequate circulation
    b. heavy bleeding
    c. difficulty breathing
    d. hypoglycemia

124. Typical changes to a woman's body during late pregnancy include:

    a. increased blood pressure.
    b. increased cardiac output.
    c. reduced heart rate.
    d. reduced blood volume.

125. Amniotic fluid is normally:

    a. greenish.
    b. brownish.
    c. clear.
    d. mixed with blood.

126. Which of the following statements regarding the first stage of labor is **FALSE**?

    a. The first stage can last up to 16 hours.
    b. The first stage may last less than 4 hours.
    c. Watery, bloody discharge may occur.
    d. Contractions last 30 seconds to 1 minute.

Questions 127 to 129 pertain to the following scenario:

> You receive a call from a panicked taxicab driver, telling you that a woman is having a baby in his cab. When you arrive, a crowd has gathered around the cab. A woman is lying in the back seat, moaning. She complains of needing to go to the bathroom.

127. The first step in caring for this patient is to
    a. allow her to go to the bathroom.
    b. tell bystanders to leave.
    c. transport the patient to the hospital.
    d. remove the patient's clothing to view the vaginal opening.

128. Bulging is visible at the vaginal opening. The patient insists that she does not want to have the baby in the cab and begs you to take her to the hospital. You should:
    a. transport the patient to the hospital.
    b. elevate the patient's buttocks with blankets or a pillow and prepare for delivery.
    c. prepare for delivery by positioning the patient with one foot on the car seat and one on the floor.
    d. time the patient's contractions.

129. In delivering the baby, you should
    a. place one hand below the baby's head.
    b. gently pull on the baby to facilitate delivery.
    c. once the head delivers, tell the mother to push.
    d. gently grasp the baby by the feet.

130. To establish that a baby is breathing, you should:
    a. hold the baby up by the feet and slap the buttocks.
    b. snap your index finger against the sole of the foot.
    c. provide supplemental oxygen by placing tubing in the baby's mouth.
    d. suction the baby's nose.

131. In delivering the placenta, you should:
    a. put pressure on the mother's abdomen over the uterus.
    b. leave afterbirth tissue within the uterus.
    c. save the afterbirth in a container.
    d. check for meconium staining.

Questions 132 to 134 pertain to the following scenario:

> The sister of an 80-year-old man reports that her brother is bleeding profusely. On arrival, the man is conscious and lying on the couch with his legs up. The seat of his pants is soaked in blood, as are the towels placed underneath. The patient states

that he is bleeding from his rectum. The bleeding began after dinner, when he felt a sharp pain in his lower abdomen.

132. Severe blood loss in an adult is defined as:

    a. 150 cc
    b. 250 cc
    c. 500 cc
    d. 1000 cc

133. To estimate the amount of blood lost, you should:

    a. pour a pint of fluid on the floor and soak a garment in it.
    b. wait for signs of hypoperfusion to appear.
    c. remove the patient's clothing.
    d. ask the patient.

134. The first line of treatment for this patient would be to:

    a. ensure an open airway.
    b. obtain a detailed history.
    c. wait for signs of hypoperfusion to appear.
    d. administer CPR.

135. A tourniquet should be used:

    a. to control external bleeding from an extremity.
    b. for joint injuries.
    c. as a last resort.
    d. to control internal bleeding from an extremity.

136. A large piece of glass becomes lodged in the eye of a bystander during a bar fight. The best line of treatment should be to:

    a. attempt to remove the piece of glass.
    b. place a paper cup over the piece of glass.
    c. assess for signs of shock.
    d. apply a bandage over the piece of glass.

137. Which of the following statements regarding a twin birth is **FALSE**?

    a. There may be a separate placenta for each baby.
    b. The second baby may deliver in a breech position.
    c. The placenta delivers only after the second twin is born.
    d. The umbilical cord of the first twin should be cut before the second twin is born.

138. In treating a woman who has miscarried, you should:

    a. save all expelled tissues.
    b. pack the vagina to absorb bleeding.
    c. replace expelled tissues in the vagina.
    d. discard any blood-soaked pads.

139. Which of the following statements regarding intubation is **FALSE**?

   a. Press on the throat to push the vocal cords into view.
   b. Air sounds should be heard in the epigastrium.
   c. Hold the tube against the patient's teeth to prevent it from moving.
   d. You may only need one hand to work the BVM.

140. Activated charcoal may be safely used in:

   a. patients with altered mental status.
   b. patients who have ingested acid.
   c. patients who have ingested gasoline.
   d. patients who have ingested aspirin.

141. The first course of treatment for a poisoning victim is:

   a. syrup of ipecac.
   b. activated charcoal.
   c. sorbitol.
   d. antidote.

Questions 142 to 144 pertain to the following scenario:

   You are called to the scene of an outdoor festival by the sister of a young woman who has been stung by a bee. The patient is sitting on the ground and is breathing rapidly. She reports nausea and her skin is flushed and blotchy. Hives are visible in the area around the sting. The patient's sister says she had an allergic reaction to a bee sting as a child.

142. The first step in treating this patient would be to:

   a. administer epinephrine.
   b. begin care for shock.
   c. administer oxygen.
   d. request an ALS intercept.

143. The patient is unable to get up and appears disoriented. She has a rapid pulse and her blood pressure is low. You should proceed by:

   a. treating for shock.
   b. administering epinephrine.
   c. administering oxygen.
   d. calling medical direction.

144. The patient's sister suddenly remembers that her sister had been prescribed epinephrine for the allergic reaction she experienced as a child. In this case, you should:

   a. treat for shock.
   b. consult medical direction and administer epinephrine.
   c. provide artificial ventilation and transport.
   d. monitor vital signs and transport.

Questions 145 to 147 pertain to the following scenario:

   On a busy city street, a 50-year-old woman has been knocked down by a bike messenger. She is conscious and sitting on the step of a building. The patient says

- 162 -

she automatically extended her right hand to break the fall. Her right wrist is bruised and swollen and her right knee joint is locked into an abnormal position. She complains of feeling "pins and needles" in her right hand.

145. The first step in treating this patient's injuries is to:

a. assess distal PMS.
b. splint.
c. realign the wrist.
d. apply a cervical collar.

146. In treating the patient's wrist injury, you should:

a. induce crepitus.
b. realign the wrist.
c. splint.
d. apply wet heat.

147. In treating the patient's knee injury, you should:

a. splint in the found position.
b. realign.
c. apply an ice pack.
d. apply wet heat.

148. Proper care of an injury to the fibula or tibia includes:

a. treating for shock.
b. applying an ice pack.
c. applying wet heat.
d. applying manual traction.

149. Which of the following statements regarding concussion is **FALSE**?

a. Concussion usually causes no detectable brain damage.
b. Concussion may be associated with amnesia.
c. Concussion may result in long-term memory loss.
d. Concussion may or may not result in loss of consciousness.

150. In removing a child from a car safety seat, you should:

a. slide the child out of the seat.
b. strap the child across the abdomen.
c. tape the child across the chin.
d. apply a cervical collar.

Answer Key and Explanations

1. B: The first step in treating a patient with potential cardiac arrest is to administer oxygen. At that point, you should obtain a patient history and perform a physical exam to obtain baseline vital signs.

2. D: When a patient loses consciousness, the first step is to open the airway. If you find the patient to be in cardiac arrest based on your initial assessment, you should attach an automated external defibrillator.

3. B: In addition to administering oxygen, the most effective way to decrease oxygen demand is to calm and reassure the patient. Driving at high speed, flashing lights, or turning on the siren will only heighten the patient's distress.

4. C: In a young child with possible airway obstruction, attempts to remove a mild obstruction may result in severe obstruction. Back blows and chest thrusts should only be performed in the case of a severe obstruction, and finger sweeps only when the child is unconscious and the object is visible in the mouth. The most appropriate course of action is to avoid agitating the child and provide immediate transport to the hospital.

5. A: Young children typically fear a stranger in their environment and will maintain eye contact with that person. Thus, inattentiveness to your presence is indicative of an altered mental state.

6. D: High fever, generalized rash, and altered mental state are indicative of meningitis, or inflammation of the tissue protecting the brain and spinal cord. Because a child with meningitis is at high risk for seizures, his or her condition should be carefully monitored during transport to the hospital.

7. C: Rapid trauma assessment is indicated in patients with significant mechanisms of injury, such as penetrating wounds to the head, neck, chest, or abdomen, falls from a height of >15 feet (such as from a tall building), or multiple long bone fractures.

8. D: In patients with acute ischemic stroke, administering oxygen is the most important first step, followed by rapid transport to the hospital for fibrinolytic therapy. Fibrinolytic therapy must be performed within 3 hours of symptom onset.

9. C: Crowning indicates that the second stage of labor has begun and delivery is imminent. After stopping the ambulance, gentle pressure should be applied to the infant's head to avoid explosive delivery.

10. B: If the umbilical cord continues to pulsate and the infant is not breathing adequately, the cord should remain attached and the head of the infant kept at the level of the mother's perineum until arrival at the hospital. The umbilical cord should not be clamped or cut until the cord has stopped pulsating and the infant has begun to breathe normally.

11. B: It may be difficult to extend the head and flex the neck of an elderly person because of arthritic conditions. The head of an elderly person should never be forced back. Rather, the jaw should be thrust forward and the tongue pulled out of the airway.

12. A: Two major risk factors for airway obstruction in elderly patients are poorly chewed food and dentures. If dentures are loose or ill-fitting and/or obstruct efforts to ventilate the patient, they should be removed.

13. C: When a patient begins to make gurgling sounds, whether before, during, or after ventilation, he or she should be suctioned immediately; however, a patient should be properly oxygenated before suctioning.

14. C: An EMT-B can help prevent future falls in an elderly patient by assessing the patient's home for potential hazards, such as slippery rugs or obstructive furniture.

15. D: Oral glucose, activated charcoal, and oxygen are carried on an ambulance and may be administered to a patient under certain circumstances.

16. A: If previously prescribed for the patient, the EMT-B may assist him or her in taking nitroglycerin, epinephrine, or inhalers. Permission from medical direction may be required.

17. B: Blood loss, trauma, particularly from abdominal injury, infection, and dehydration resulting from diarrhea or vomiting are the most common causes of hypoperfusion in infants and children. Bleeding that may not seem serious in an adult may lead to hypoperfusion in a child.

18. C: Signs of hypoperfusion in a child include rapid respiratory rate, pale, clammy skin, weak or absent peripheral pulse, and decreased urinary output.

19. D: Because infants and children may go into decompensated shock rapidly, never wait for signs of decompensated shock to develop. Supplemental oxygen should be provided, external bleeding managed, and artificial ventilation begun if necessary. The child should be kept warm and transported immediately to the hospital.

20. A: Although a cardiac condition is the most likely cause of cardiac arrest in adults, respiratory failure is the most likely cause in children. Breathing difficulties in children may result from airway obstruction or respiratory disease.

21. C: Because the patient has been lying in the cold all night, he is most likely suffering from hypothermia. Signs of hypothermia include muscular rigidity, amnesia, and loss of contact with environment.

22. D: The best course of action to prevent additional body heat loss in an injured patient trapped in cold environment is to create a barrier to the cold. Blankets or articles of clothing can be used to protect the patient from exposure to wind or water. Active rewarming may result in cardiac arrest, and ingestion of stimulants in impaired circulation.

23. A: Individuals under the influence of alcohol or drugs may be more susceptible to hypothermia. The fact that the patient had been drinking and was trapped overnight in a cold environment places him at high risk of hypothermia.

24. B: The signs and symptoms of carbon monoxide poisoning may resemble those of the flu, including nausea and headache.

25. A: The first step in treating a patient with an absorbed poison is to remove the poison from the eyes or skin immediately. This may be accomplished by irrigating the eye or skin with clean water for 20 minutes. Attempting to neutralize the absorbed substance with other solutions such as vinegar or baking soda may make the injury worse.

- 165 -

26. B: Other conditions such as diabetes, epilepsy, and hypoxia may produce symptoms resembling those of alcohol intoxication. Given that the patient has hit his head, his symptoms could be due to head injury.

27. A: Because intoxicated patients could also be suffering from a medical emergency or an injury, they should be transported to the hospital for further assessment. Patients with even minor head injuries may be prone to subdural hematoma. Asking the patient if he has taken drugs may provoke a violent reaction; however, calling law enforcement without properly assessing the patient's condition may result in serious adverse events or even death.

28. C: Substance or alcohol abusers may appear calm and then suddenly become violent. For your own protection, if the situation becomes unsafe and you have not been trained in law enforcement, you should immediately leave the scene and call the police for assistance.

29. D: Breath sounds should always be heard bilaterally. If breath sounds are absent on the left but present on the right, the endotracheal tube has been incorrectly inserted into the right bronchus. If breath sounds are only present in the epigastrium, the esophagus has been intubated, which may result in a life-threatening condition.

30. D: The accuracy of an oximeter reading may be affected in patients in shock or with hypothermia because low body temperature restricts blood flow through the capillaries. Carbon monoxide poisoning produces falsely high readings; because cigarettes produce carbon monoxide, chronic smokers may also have falsely high readings.

31. A: SAMPLE stands for the elements of a patient's history, including signs and symptoms, past medical history, and use of medications. It is always important to obtain a patient's medication history, especially in the case of an older patient.

32. B: Sweating is an example of a vital sign. Taking a patient's vital signs and symptoms is the first step in obtaining a SAMPLE history.

33. C: Nitroglycerin is usually prescribed for patients with angina pectoris, or chest pain.

34. D: Compared with adults, infants and children have a faster pulse and respiratory rate and lower blood pressure.

35. C: Oral requests from a family member are not sufficient reason to withhold care. If a legal DNR (Do Not Resuscitate) order is not presented, an EMT-B is obligated to provide care.

36. B: In some states, an off-duty EMT-B has no legal obligation to provide care; however, you may feel a moral obligation to help a patient in need. It is always best to provide care and contact other emergency personnel for additional help. Leaving the scene of an accident, even after providing care, may be construed as abandoning a patient.

37. C: Mental status, condition of the airway, breathing, and circulation should be assessed in all patients, whether responsive or unresponsive, and with either trauma or a medical condition. Capillary refill is used to assess infants and children only.

38. B: The normal pulse rate for an adult is between 60 and 100 beats per minute. In an emergency situation, the pulse rate may rise to between 100 and 140 beats per minute. A pulse rate below 50 beats per minute indicates a serious problem.

39. D: A high pulse in a child is usually not a cause for concern; however, a low pulse may be indicative of imminent cardiac arrest.

40. C: Because your thumb has its own pulse, you should not use it to take someone else's pulse. Applying too much pressure can press the artery shut. The carotid pulse should not be assessed on both sides at the same time; rather, if you have difficulty finding a pulse on one side, try the other side.

41. B: Soft-tissue trauma to the head, face, or neck is indicative of cervical spine injury.

42. A: In the case of a potential cervical spine injury, you should immediately stabilize the patient's head and neck manually. The head and neck should be stabilized until he or she is completely immobilized and secured to a backboard.

43. B: In the case of possible cervical spine injury, a rigid collar should be applied before transporting the patient to the hospital; a soft collar is not sufficient to immobilize the cervical spine. The patient's head should be kept in a neutral position, not turned to one side or tilted front or back. Once the collar is in place, the back of the neck cannot be palpated.

44. C: A detailed physical exam is most often performed on a trauma patient with a significant mechanism of injury rather than a patient with no significant injury or a medical patient.

45. D: Oxygen should never be withheld from a patient in respiratory distress, even those with a chronic lung disease such as bronchitis or emphysema.

46. C: Gurgling sounds usually indicate the presence of fluid in the throat.

47. B: COPD patients with difficulty breathing are typically in the tripod position, leaning forward with hands on knees.

48. C: Altered mental status in a patient with breathing difficulty usually indicates a lack of oxygen. If the patient is not breathing adequately, artificial ventilation should be performed and supplemental oxygen should be provided.

49. D: Never rub or squeeze a frostbitten or frozen area, as this can seriously damage the injured tissue. Active rewarming is seldom recommended in cases of frostbite or freezing because of the risk of permanent injury. You should administer high-concentration oxygen, cover the frozen or frostbitten area, and transport the patient to the hospital immediately.

50. B: If transport is delayed and the local protocol recommends it, begin active rewarming of the frozen area, taking care that the injured area does not touch the sides or bottom of the container. Never massage or rub snow on a frostbitten or frozen area. Patients should not be allowed to smoke or drink alcoholic beverages because of the risk of decreasing circulation.

51. C: During the course of active rewarming, keep the affected area immersed until the water cools, even if the patient complains of pain, then remove the affected part and add more warm water; complaints of moderate or even intense pain indicate that rewarming has been successful. Do not apply pressure or allow the patient to walk on the affected area. Once rewarming has been completed, apply a dry sterile dressing to the affected area and cover with blankets, but do not allow the blanket to come into contact with the injured area.

52. B: In the case of a near-drowning, rescue breathing should be initiated without delay, even if the victim is still in the water. Chest compression is only effective when the victim is out of the water.

53. A: Never attempt to suck the venom from a snakebite. Do not put ice on the bite unless instructed to do so by a physician or local protocol. The bite should be cleaned with soap and water and the patient transported to the hospital immediately.

54. B: Typical signs and symptoms in a heat emergency patient with hot and dry or moist skin include little or no perspiration, full and rapid pulse, and seizures but not muscle cramps.

55. D: Typical signs and symptoms of a heat emergency patient with normal or cool moist, pale skin include muscle cramps, heavy perspiration, and weak pulse rate.

56. B: Diabetes or low blood sugar can produce symptoms--such as hostile behavior, drooling, heavy perspiration, or seizures--that mimic those of a psychiatric condition.

57. D: The best approach in treating a hostile or aggressive patient is to watch for sudden changes in behavior and seek assistance from law enforcement. Restraining the patient or forcing him or her to accept emergency care is usually not in the legal jurisdiction of an EMT-B.

58. C: Soft restraints such as leather cuffs or belts are acceptable means of restraint for violent patients; handcuffs or plastic "throwaway" restraints may cause soft tissue damage. "Hog-tying" can impair breathing and result in positional asphyxia.

59. D: Never place an object such as a thermometer, tongue blade, or oral airway into the mouth of a child with epiglottitis, as this could obstruct the airway. The child should not be forced to lie down, which may be uncomfortable, but should be transported to the hospital in a sitting position on his or her parent's lap.

60. B: Do not use rubbing alcohol to reduce the child's temperature, because it can be toxic if absorbed in high amounts. Submerging the child in cold water or applying cold towels can result in hypothermia. The child should be transported to the hospital as soon as possible.

61. B: The best line of treatment for a child with diarrhea and vomiting is to maintain an open airway and administer oxygen. Oral suctioning may be required for vomiting. Sipping water or ice chips is usually recommended for children with diarrhea only.

62. C: The first step in assessing a child with fever is to obtain a relative skin temperature using a skin thermometer or by applying the back of your hand to the child's forehead or abdomen. Oral or rectal temperatures are generally not taken in the prehospital setting.

63. A: If a child has a seizure on transport, you should maintain an open airway and administer oxygen. Never insert an oropharyngeal airway or a bite stick. Seizures caused by fever should always be considered life-threatening.

64. D: Consuming even small amounts of iron can be life-threatening in children. Usual signs of iron poisoning include nausea, diarrhea, and bloody vomiting.

65. C: Because meningitis is an airborne disease, a surgical mask should always be worn when caring for a child with suspected meningitis. An EMT-B with possible exposure to meningitis should be evaluated by a physician as soon as possible.

66. A: Sounding the siren when close to another vehicle can result in the driver panicking and jamming on his brakes; use the horn to alert the driver instead. Continuous use of a siren can make motorists less likely to yield the right of way, can increase stress and anxiety in injured or ill patients, and has been associated with increased operator driving speed.

67. C: An emergency vehicle is allowed to pass in a no-passing zone, exceed the speed limit, and pass through a stop sign as long as it is safe to do so; however, in the case of a school bus with blinking red lights, the operator of the vehicle should wait for the bus driver to clear the children and turn off the red lights.

68. B: Four-way flashers or directional signals should not be used as emergency lights because they can confuse other drivers.

69. C: Highly traumatized patients should be transported to the hospital as soon as possible; spending too much time packaging a patient in this condition can result in death. In some cases, the patient must be moved before emergency care is completed. Sheets and blankets should be tucked under the mattress and stretcher and the patient secured to a spine board or other patient-carrying device.

70. B: Vital signs should be assessed every 5 minutes in an unstable patient and every 15 minutes in a stable patient.

71. A: A non-emergency patient should never be left alone; an EMT-B should remain with the patient at all times. In cases when the emergency department is especially busy, the patient can remain in the ambulance until the operator decides where he or she should be taken.

72. B: Although a vehicle that is upright on all four wheels appears stable, it can be rocked forward or backward or side to side, possibly injuring those inside; the tires of an upright vehicle should always be deflated during stabilization. When placing cribbing, you should never kneel down; maintain a squatting position on both feet to move quickly in case the car moves suddenly. Stabilization is unnecessary only in the case of a car with its roof crushed flat against the body.

73. A: Always make sure the patient has been decontaminated before transporting him or her to the hospital; a contaminated patient or EMT-B can contaminate the entire ambulance team. If a patient requires immediate life-saving care, even if he or she has not been decontaminated, you should provide that care, being careful to wear protective clothing and to decontaminate yourself as soon as possible.

74. D: A patient in cardiac arrest is considered Priority 4 or 0 because immediate treatment in such a patient is not justified when many other individuals need attention; however, such patients can be upgraded to Priority 1 when ample resources become available.

75. B: In the case of an accident involving multiple casualties, an ambulance should not transport patients without approval of the transportation officer; failure to comply with the directions of a transportation officer could result in patients being taken to the wrong treatment facility.

76. C: In a child, the tongue is larger, the chest wall is softer, and the trachea is narrower compared with those of an adult.

77. A: Seesaw breathing, in which the chest and abdomen move in opposite directions, often occurs in children but not adults with inadequate breathing.

78. C: Orotracheal intubation may stimulate the airway, resulting in slowing of the heart rate.

79. A: In the case of an infiltrated IV, the needle has either punctured the vein and exited the other side or pulled out of the vein entirely, resulting in fluid flowing into the surrounding tissue. The IV flow should be stopped and the IV discontinued.

80. D: Signs or symptoms indicative of an acute psychological problem following a stressful event include uncontrollable crying, inappropriate behavior, or irrational thoughts; however, nausea, loss of appetite, or difficulty sleeping are typical reactions and usually do not require intervention.

81. B: The first step in assessing an adult patient who has collapsed is to determine responsiveness. This can be done by gently tapping the patient and asking, "Are you OK?" If the patient is able to respond, resuscitation is unnecessary.

82. A: The first step in treating an unconscious child or infant is to resuscitate for 1 minute, then activate EMS.

83. B: To determine the pulse of an adult or a child, you should feel for the carotid artery; feel for the brachial artery in infants.

84. C: If the patient has a pulse, chest compression is not required. If the patient is not breathing, provide artificial ventilation; if the patient has stopped breathing and has no pulse, begin CPR.

85. D: The jaw-thrust maneuver is the only recommended procedure for opening the airway in an unconscious patient with a possible spinal injury.

86. B: Rescue breathing can blow air into the patient's stomach, causing distention. In the case of gastric distention and vomiting, roll the patient onto his or her side. Simply turning the patient's head can lead to aspiration of vomitus or aggravation of spinal injury.

87. A: When releasing chest compression, you should straighten your arms, lock your elbows, and keep your hands on the patient's sternum. Move from the hips, which should act as a fulcrum.

88. D: Tendons connect muscles to bones.

89. C: A laceration may not seem to be serious, but can result in severe infection or scarring if not treated properly. The patient's pulse should be checked, as well as motor and sensory function distal to the injury.

90. D: Never try to remove an impaled object; twisting or putting pressure on the object can cause additional injury. Instead, stabilize the object by applying a bulky dressing.

91. C: The avulsed body part should be saved by wrapping it in a dry sterile dressing and then placing it in a plastic bag, plastic wrap, or aluminum foil. Do not place the part in dry ice, water, or saline.

92. A: Contrary to popular belief, a gunshot wound to the abdomen without an exit wound may still cause serious injury. Bullets can be deflected or explode, sending out pieces that can injure adjacent areas of the body.

93. D: Although burns caused by electrical current may result in relatively minor skin injury, they can present a high risk of severe internal injury.

94. B: Compared with that of an adult, an infant's head is larger in proportion to the rest of the body; thus, while an adult's head accounts for 9% of body surface area, an infant's head accounts for 18%.

95. C: Burns caused by hydrofluoric acid, a chemical commonly used in manufacturing, should be flushed with water as soon as possible.

96. C: In treating a chemical burn to the eye, immediately flood the eye with water; continue washing the eye during transport for at least 20 minutes or until arrival at the hospital. Do not use vinegar or baking soda to neutralize the chemical.

97. B: In bandaging an open wound, take care not to bandage too tightly or too loosely and do not leave loose ends. Fingers and toes should remain exposed to observe changes in circulation unless they have been burned; in that case, they should be covered.

98. B: Patients with treatable injuries that may be life-threatening such as airway or breathing difficulties should be classified as Priority 1 and treated first.

99. B: A patient who has gone into cardiac arrest should be classified as Priority 4 or 0; these patients should not receive treatment unless none of the other patients are at risk of dying or sustaining long-term disability if left untreated.

100. C: Patients with back injuries with or without spinal cord damage should be classified as Priority 2.

101. C: The correct sequence of connective function is muscle-tendon-bone and bone-ligament-bone.

102. B: A dramatic injury to the extremity such as a protruding bone should not distract you from assessing an accident victim for life-threatening injury, such as a spinal fracture. Multiple fractures, particularly to the femur, can result in life-threatening external or internal bleeding.

103. A: In the case of a deformity such as a protruding bone, you should realign the injury to its correct anatomical position and splint; splinting the deformed part in its original position may worsen the injury.

104. C: Femur fractures often cause spasm of the large muscle groups of the thigh, resulting in severe pain and further soft-tissue injury; for this reason, a traction splint should be used to counteract muscle spasm and reduce pain.

105. D: The best method of care for an open abdominal injury is to apply a sterile saline dressing over the wound, then apply an occlusive dressing. Never give the patient something by mouth or touch or replace an exposed or eviscerated organ; use of an aluminum foil occlusive dressing may cut an eviscerated organ.

106. A: Sometimes a dislocated shoulder will go back into place on its own; never attempt to straighten out a dislocation. A rigid splint should not be used for shoulder injuries. In the case of a possible cervical spine injury, do not tie a sling around the patient's neck.

107. B: A hip fracture is a fracture of the proximal femur, not the pelvis.

108. D: In treating an ankle or foot injury, stabilize the limb, taking care not to change the position of the ankle, and tie a pillow to the ankle and foot. Do not apply manual traction or put an ice pack directly on the skin.

109. C: The pneumatic anti-shock garment (PASG) is indicated in cases of bleeding, pelvic injury, or abdominal trauma; it is contraindicated in patients with cardiogenic shock or shock in the presence of a chest wound.

110. B: A blood glucose meter reading above 120 or 140, depending on the manufacturer, indicates hyperglycemia; a reading below 80 indicates hypoglycemia.

111. A: Diabetic children are at increased risk of a medical emergency compared with diabetic adults.

112. B: Under the Ryan White act, in the case of possible exposure of an EMT to the bodily fluids of a patient with possible bloodborne disease, a hospital is only required to review the patient's medical records for evidence of bloodborne disease. Hospitals cannot test a patient for bloodborne disease simply at the request of an EMT or designated officer.

113. D: Children or mentally incompetent adults cannot legally refuse treatment; however, care can be given to a child without parental consent in the case of life-threatening illness or injury when the parent or guardian is not present.

114. C: Patient information cannot be disclosed based on verbal permission or over the telephone but only if the patient has signed a written release; however, patient information can be discussed with healthcare personnel caring for the patient, such as a doctor or nurse.

115. A: A supine patient is lying on his or her back; a prone patient is lying on his or her abdomen, and a patient lying on his or her side is in the recovery position.

116. C: In the Trendelenburg position, the patient lies with the head slightly lower than the feet; this position is often used to treat patients in shock.

117. D: A fractured rib can cause inadequate breathing and thus be life-threatening.

118. B: The preferred method for moving a patient down stairs is to use a stair chair or wheeled stretcher; this method is usually safer and more efficient.

119. A: When immediate care is necessary, urgent moves may be used to move a patient with spinal injury; however, precautions must be made to avoid further spinal injury. The extremity lift, direct carry, and draw-sheet methods are only used to move patients with no suspected spinal injury.

120. B: Never park the ambulance in the danger zone; the ambulance should be parked away from broken glass or other debris.

121. C: As part of the initial assessment of an accident or crime scene, you should take the necessary body substance isolation (BSI) precautions to avoid exposure to the patient's blood, saliva, and other body fluids. BSI precautions include wearing gloves, protective eyewear, and/or a protective mask when providing patient care.

122. B: In the case of an accident, no matter how minor, always identify the mechanism of injury, determine what injuries are possible, and treat the patient accordingly. Never assume that there are no injuries, even if the patient claims he or she is unhurt. In the case of the driver who was thrown against the wheel, although no signs of bruising or other injury are apparent, he may have sustained blunt-force trauma and should be treated accordingly.

123. D: Inadequate circulation, blood loss, and difficulty breathing are all signs of a life-threatening condition.

124. B: Typical body changes during the last trimester include increases in heart rate, blood volume, and cardiac output; blood pressure usually decreases slightly.

125. C: Normally, amniotic fluid is clear; a greenish or brownish color may indicate maternal or fetal distress. Bleeding does not accompany breakage of the amniotic sac.

126. D: The first stage of labor can be as long as 16 hours or as short as 4 hours and is usually associated with watery, bloody discharge. Contractions lasting 30 seconds to 1 minute indicate that delivery is imminent.

127. B: Your first step is to protect the patient from staring bystanders, asking them to leave in a polite but firm manner. Next, you should help the patient to remove any clothing that obstructs your view of the vaginal opening. A feeling of an impending bowel movement and bulging at the vaginal opening indicate that birth is imminent; however, the patient should not be allowed to use the bathroom. Because the baby may be born any minute, transport is not practical at this time.

128. C: Visible bulging at the vaginal opening indicates that crowning is taking place and that birth is imminent. At this point, it is not practical to transport the patient; instead, you should gently position the mother in the cab with one foot resting on the seat and the other on the floor and prepare for delivery.

129. A: The baby should be supported throughout the entire birth process. Place one hand below the baby's head as it delivers. Tell the mother not to push while you check to make sure the umbilical cord is not wrapped around the baby's neck. Never pull on the baby during delivery; grasping a slippery baby by the feet may cause you to drop the child.

130. B: Assess breathing by snapping your index finger against the sole of the baby's foot. Contrary to popular belief, you should not hold the baby by the feet and slap the buttocks. If supplemental oxygen is needed, place tubing close to but not into the baby's mouth. Suction the baby's mouth first to prevent aspiration of blood, fluids, or other materials into the lungs.

131. C: In delivering the placenta or afterbirth, remember that the process can take 20 to 30 minutes. Do not place pressure on the mother's abdomen. Once the placenta delivers, do not leave any afterbirth tissues in the vagina because of the risk of infection; save the afterbirth in a container and give it to the attending physician on arrival at the hospital.

132. D: In an adult, sudden blood loss of 1000 cc or 1 liter is considered serious; however, because children have a lower blood volume compared with adults, blood loss of 500 cc is considered serious in a child. Blood loss of 150 cc would be serious in an infant.

133. A: Although it is difficult to estimate blood loss, a useful method is to pour a pint of liquid on the floor and soak a garment in it to observe how wet it looks and feels. In a patient with blood loss, do not wait for signs of hypoperfusion or shock to develop to begin treatment.

134. A: In this case, bleeding from the rectum is a sign of internal bleeding, which may rapidly lead to hypoperfusion or shock. In cases of suspected internal bleeding, the first step should be to ensure an open airway and assess breathing and circulation. Do not wait for signs of shock to appear before beginning treatment.

135. C: A tourniquet may cause serious injury to the nerves, muscles, or blood vessels and may result in loss of a limb; for this reason, it should only be used as a last resort in cases of life-threatening bleeding.

136. B: The best line of treatment for an object impaled in the eye such as a piece of glass is to place a roll of 3-inch gauze bandage on each side of the object to stabilize it, then place a paper cup over

the object and allow it to rest on the rolls of gauze. Do not place a bandage directly over the object or the cup.

137. C: In a twin birth, the placenta may deliver either before or after the birth of the second twin. There may be a separate placenta for each baby or a single one for both. Breech birth is common in the second twin; the umbilical cord of the first twin should be tied or cut before the birth of the second twin.

138. A: In the case of a miscarriage, always save the expelled tissues but do not attempt to replace or remove them from the vagina. Blood-soaked pads should also be replaced and saved. Do not pack the vagina.

139. B: Air sounds in the epigastrium indicate that the tube has been incorrectly placed in the esophagus; the tube should then be removed and the process repeated. You may need to press on the patient's throat to view the vocal cords in order to maneuver the tube correctly. The tube should be held against the patient's teeth to ensure that it does not move. You may not necessarily need two hands to work the bag-valve-mask unit (BVM) because the patient will be less resistant to ventilation.

140. D: Activated charcoal is contraindicated in patients who have ingested acids or alkalis, such as those found in bathroom or oven cleaners, in patients who have ingested gasoline during siphoning, and in those with altered mental status.

141. B: Activated charcoal is the preferred line of treatment for a poisoning victim and is superior to syrup of ipecac in speed and effectiveness. Only a few antidotes exist for a relatively small number of poisons. Because sorbitol acts very quickly, it is not usually given for poisoning in most EMS situations.

142. C: The first step in treating a patient with a severe allergic reaction is to manage the patient's airway and breathing. Administer high-concentration oxygen; if the patient has difficulty breathing, provide artificial ventilation. If the patient exhibits signs of shock such as altered mental status and has a prescribed epinephrine auto-injector, you should consult medical direction and if advised, administer the epinephrine; if the patient shows signs of shock but has not been prescribed epinephrine, you should treat for shock and transport immediately.

143. A: In the case of a patient who has had an allergic reaction in the past but has not been prescribed epinephrine and exhibits signs of shock such as altered mental status, increased pulse, reduced blood pressure, and nausea or vomiting, you should treat for shock and transport immediately.

144. B: If the patient exhibits signs of shock and has been prescribed an epinephrine auto-injector, you should call medical direction and if advised, administer epinephrine. If the patient does not have the auto-injector with them, you may request an advanced life support (ALS) intercept; paramedics carry and can administer epinephrine.

145. A: Musculoskeletal injuries carry the risk of nerve and blood vessel injury; for this reason, you should assess distal pulse, motor function, and sensation (PMS) before splinting.

146. C: Patients with a painful, swollen, or deformed extremity should be treated for possible fracture. After assessing distal PMS, you should splint the wrist, then reassess. Check for nerve injury by asking the patient if he or she can move the injured part or feel your touch. Never induce

crepitus, a grating sound or feeling that causes severe pain. Realignment is unnecessary unless the hand is cyanotic or lacks pulses.

147. A: A joint locked in a normal or abnormal position may be dislocated. Joint injuries should usually be splinted in the direction in which they were found; in the case of an angulated injury to the ulna, femur, or radius that cannot fit into a rigid splint, you should realign the bone.

148. A: A patient with an injury to the tibia or fibula should be treated for shock. Administer high-concentration oxygen and splint the injury. Do not apply manual traction, or tension, and do not apply an ice pack directly to the skin.

149. C: Concussion may result in amnesia, or short-term loss of memory of the events surrounding the accident; however, concussion rarely results in long-term memory loss.

150. D: In removing an injured child from a car safety seat, apply a cervical collar to maintain manual stabilization of the head and neck. Do not slide the child out of the seat or strap the child to the backboard across the abdomen. Taping the child across the chin may put pressure on the neck.

How to Overcome Test Anxiety

Just the thought of taking a test is enough to make most people a little nervous. A test is an important event that can have a long-term impact on your future, so it's important to take it seriously and it's natural to feel anxious about performing well. But just because anxiety is normal, that doesn't mean that it's helpful in test taking, or that you should simply accept it as part of your life. Anxiety can have a variety of effects. These effects can be mild, like making you feel slightly nervous, or severe, like blocking your ability to focus or remember even a simple detail.

If you experience test anxiety—whether severe or mild—it's important to know how to beat it. To discover this, first you need to understand what causes test anxiety.

Causes of Test Anxiety

While we often think of anxiety as an uncontrollable emotional state, it can actually be caused by simple, practical things. One of the most common causes of test anxiety is that a person does not feel adequately prepared for their test. This feeling can be the result of many different issues such as poor study habits or lack of organization, but the most common culprit is time management. Starting to study too late, failing to organize your study time to cover all of the material, or being distracted while you study will mean that you're not well prepared for the test. This may lead to cramming the night before, which will cause you to be physically and mentally exhausted for the test. Poor time management also contributes to feelings of stress, fear, and hopelessness as you realize you are not well prepared but don't know what to do about it.

Other times, test anxiety is not related to your preparation for the test but comes from unresolved fear. This may be a past failure on a test, or poor performance on tests in general. It may come from comparing yourself to others who seem to be performing better or from the stress of living up to expectations. Anxiety may be driven by fears of the future—how failure on this test would affect your educational and career goals. These fears are often completely irrational, but they can still negatively impact your test performance.

> **Review Video:** 3 Reasons You Have Test Anxiety
> Visit mometrix.com/academy and enter code: 428468

Elements of Test Anxiety

As mentioned earlier, test anxiety is considered to be an emotional state, but it has physical and mental components as well. Sometimes you may not even realize that you are suffering from test anxiety until you notice the physical symptoms. These can include trembling hands, rapid heartbeat, sweating, nausea, and tense muscles. Extreme anxiety may lead to fainting or vomiting. Obviously, any of these symptoms can have a negative impact on testing. It is important to recognize them as soon as they begin to occur so that you can address the problem before it damages your performance.

> **Review Video:** <u>3 Ways to Tell You Have Test Anxiety</u>
> Visit mometrix.com/academy and enter code: 927847

The mental components of test anxiety include trouble focusing and inability to remember learned information. During a test, your mind is on high alert, which can help you recall information and stay focused for an extended period of time. However, anxiety interferes with your mind's natural processes, causing you to blank out, even on the questions you know well. The strain of testing during anxiety makes it difficult to stay focused, especially on a test that may take several hours. Extreme anxiety can take a huge mental toll, making it difficult not only to recall test information but even to understand the test questions or pull your thoughts together.

> **Review Video:** <u>How Test Anxiety Affects Memory</u>
> Visit mometrix.com/academy and enter code: 609003

Effects of Test Anxiety

Test anxiety is like a disease—if left untreated, it will get progressively worse. Anxiety leads to poor performance, and this reinforces the feelings of fear and failure, which in turn lead to poor performances on subsequent tests. It can grow from a mild nervousness to a crippling condition. If allowed to progress, test anxiety can have a big impact on your schooling, and consequently on your future.

Test anxiety can spread to other parts of your life. Anxiety on tests can become anxiety in any stressful situation, and blanking on a test can turn into panicking in a job situation. But fortunately, you don't have to let anxiety rule your testing and determine your grades. There are a number of relatively simple steps you can take to move past anxiety and function normally on a test and in the rest of life.

> **Review Video:** <u>How Test Anxiety Impacts Your Grades</u>
> Visit mometrix.com/academy and enter code: 939819

Physical Steps for Beating Test Anxiety

While test anxiety is a serious problem, the good news is that it can be overcome. It doesn't have to control your ability to think and remember information. While it may take time, you can begin taking steps today to beat anxiety.

Just as your first hint that you may be struggling with anxiety comes from the physical symptoms, the first step to treating it is also physical. Rest is crucial for having a clear, strong mind. If you are tired, it is much easier to give in to anxiety. But if you establish good sleep habits, your body and mind will be ready to perform optimally, without the strain of exhaustion. Additionally, sleeping well helps you to retain information better, so you're more likely to recall the answers when you see the test questions.

Getting good sleep means more than going to bed on time. It's important to allow your brain time to relax. Take study breaks from time to time so it doesn't get overworked, and don't study right before bed. Take time to rest your mind before trying to rest your body, or you may find it difficult to fall asleep.

> **Review Video: The Importance of Sleep for Your Brain**
> Visit mometrix.com/academy and enter code: 319338

Along with sleep, other aspects of physical health are important in preparing for a test. Good nutrition is vital for good brain function. Sugary foods and drinks may give a burst of energy but this burst is followed by a crash, both physically and emotionally. Instead, fuel your body with protein and vitamin-rich foods.

Also, drink plenty of water. Dehydration can lead to headaches and exhaustion, especially if your brain is already under stress from the rigors of the test. Particularly if your test is a long one, drink water during the breaks. And if possible, take an energy-boosting snack to eat between sections.

> **Review Video: How Diet Can Affect your Mood**
> Visit mometrix.com/academy and enter code: 624317

Along with sleep and diet, a third important part of physical health is exercise. Maintaining a steady workout schedule is helpful, but even taking 5-minute study breaks to walk can help get your blood pumping faster and clear your head. Exercise also releases endorphins, which contribute to a positive feeling and can help combat test anxiety.

When you nurture your physical health, you are also contributing to your mental health. If your body is healthy, your mind is much more likely to be healthy as well. So take time to rest, nourish your body with healthy food and water, and get moving as much as possible. Taking these physical steps will make you stronger and more able to take the mental steps necessary to overcome test anxiety.

> **Review Video: How to Stay Healthy and Prevent Test Anxiety**
> Visit mometrix.com/academy and enter code: 877894

Mental Steps for Beating Test Anxiety

Working on the mental side of test anxiety can be more challenging, but as with the physical side, there are clear steps you can take to overcome it. As mentioned earlier, test anxiety often stems from lack of preparation, so the obvious solution is to prepare for the test. Effective studying may be the most important weapon you have for beating test anxiety, but you can and should employ several other mental tools to combat fear.

First, boost your confidence by reminding yourself of past success—tests or projects that you aced. If you're putting as much effort into preparing for this test as you did for those, there's no reason you should expect to fail here. Work hard to prepare; then trust your preparation.

Second, surround yourself with encouraging people. It can be helpful to find a study group, but be sure that the people you're around will encourage a positive attitude. If you spend time with others who are anxious or cynical, this will only contribute to your own anxiety. Look for others who are motivated to study hard from a desire to succeed, not from a fear of failure.

Third, reward yourself. A test is physically and mentally tiring, even without anxiety, and it can be helpful to have something to look forward to. Plan an activity following the test, regardless of the outcome, such as going to a movie or getting ice cream.

When you are taking the test, if you find yourself beginning to feel anxious, remind yourself that you know the material. Visualize successfully completing the test. Then take a few deep, relaxing breaths and return to it. Work through the questions carefully but with confidence, knowing that you are capable of succeeding.

Developing a healthy mental approach to test taking will also aid in other areas of life. Test anxiety affects more than just the actual test—it can be damaging to your mental health and even contribute to depression. It's important to beat test anxiety before it becomes a problem for more than testing.

Review Video: Test Anxiety and Depression
Visit mometrix.com/academy and enter code: 904704

Study Strategy

Being prepared for the test is necessary to combat anxiety, but what does being prepared look like? You may study for hours on end and still not feel prepared. What you need is a strategy for test prep. The next few pages outline our recommended steps to help you plan out and conquer the challenge of preparation.

Step 1: Scope Out the Test

Learn everything you can about the format (multiple choice, essay, etc.) and what will be on the test. Gather any study materials, course outlines, or sample exams that may be available. Not only will this help you to prepare, but knowing what to expect can help to alleviate test anxiety.

Step 2: Map Out the Material

Look through the textbook or study guide and make note of how many chapters or sections it has. Then divide these over the time you have. For example, if a book has 15 chapters and you have five days to study, you need to cover three chapters each day. Even better, if you have the time, leave an extra day at the end for overall review after you have gone through the material in depth.

If time is limited, you may need to prioritize the material. Look through it and make note of which sections you think you already have a good grasp on, and which need review. While you are studying, skim quickly through the familiar sections and take more time on the challenging parts. Write out your plan so you don't get lost as you go. Having a written plan also helps you feel more in control of the study, so anxiety is less likely to arise from feeling overwhelmed at the amount to cover.

Step 3: Gather Your Tools

Decide what study method works best for you. Do you prefer to highlight in the book as you study and then go back over the highlighted portions? Or do you type out notes of the important information? Or is it helpful to make flashcards that you can carry with you? Assemble the pens, index cards, highlighters, post-it notes, and any other materials you may need so you won't be distracted by getting up to find things while you study.

If you're having a hard time retaining the information or organizing your notes, experiment with different methods. For example, try color-coding by subject with colored pens, highlighters, or post-it notes. If you learn better by hearing, try recording yourself reading your notes so you can listen while in the car, working out, or simply sitting at your desk. Ask a friend to quiz you from your flashcards, or try teaching someone the material to solidify it in your mind.

Step 4: Create Your Environment

It's important to avoid distractions while you study. This includes both the obvious distractions like visitors and the subtle distractions like an uncomfortable chair (or a too-comfortable couch that makes you want to fall asleep). Set up the best study environment possible: good lighting and a comfortable work area. If background music helps you focus, you may want to turn it on, but otherwise keep the room quiet. If you are using a computer to take notes, be sure you don't have any other windows open, especially applications like social media, games, or anything else that could distract you. Silence your phone and turn off notifications. Be sure to keep water close by so you stay hydrated while you study (but avoid unhealthy drinks and snacks).

Also, take into account the best time of day to study. Are you freshest first thing in the morning? Try to set aside some time then to work through the material. Is your mind clearer in the afternoon or evening? Schedule your study session then. Another method is to study at the same time of day that you will take the test, so that your brain gets used to working on the material at that time and will be ready to focus at test time.

Step 5: Study!

Once you have done all the study preparation, it's time to settle into the actual studying. Sit down, take a few moments to settle your mind so you can focus, and begin to follow your study plan. Don't give in to distractions or let yourself procrastinate. This is your time to prepare so you'll be ready to fearlessly approach the test. Make the most of the time and stay focused.

Of course, you don't want to burn out. If you study too long you may find that you're not retaining the information very well. Take regular study breaks. For example, taking five minutes out of every hour to walk briskly, breathing deeply and swinging your arms, can help your mind stay fresh.

As you get to the end of each chapter or section, it's a good idea to do a quick review. Remind yourself of what you learned and work on any difficult parts. When you feel that you've mastered the material, move on to the next part. At the end of your study session, briefly skim through your notes again.

But while review is helpful, cramming last minute is NOT. If at all possible, work ahead so that you won't need to fit all your study into the last day. Cramming overloads your brain with more information than it can process and retain, and your tired mind may struggle to recall even previously learned information when it is overwhelmed with last-minute study. Also, the urgent nature of cramming and the stress placed on your brain contribute to anxiety. You'll be more likely to go to the test feeling unprepared and having trouble thinking clearly.

So don't cram, and don't stay up late before the test, even just to review your notes at a leisurely pace. Your brain needs rest more than it needs to go over the information again. In fact, plan to finish your studies by noon or early afternoon the day before the test. Give your brain the rest of the day to relax or focus on other things, and get a good night's sleep. Then you will be fresh for the test and better able to recall what you've studied.

Step 6: Take a practice test

Many courses offer sample tests, either online or in the study materials. This is an excellent resource to check whether you have mastered the material, as well as to prepare for the test format and environment.

Check the test format ahead of time: the number of questions, the type (multiple choice, free response, etc.), and the time limit. Then create a plan for working through them. For example, if you have 30 minutes to take a 60-question test, your limit is 30 seconds per question. Spend less time on the questions you know well so that you can take more time on the difficult ones.

If you have time to take several practice tests, take the first one open book, with no time limit. Work through the questions at your own pace and make sure you fully understand them. Gradually work up to taking a test under test conditions: sit at a desk with all study materials put away and set a timer. Pace yourself to make sure you finish the test with time to spare and go back to check your answers if you have time.

After each test, check your answers. On the questions you missed, be sure you understand why you missed them. Did you misread the question (tests can use tricky wording)? Did you forget the information? Or was it something you hadn't learned? Go back and study any shaky areas that the practice tests reveal.

Taking these tests not only helps with your grade, but also aids in combating test anxiety. If you're already used to the test conditions, you're less likely to worry about it, and working through tests until you're scoring well gives you a confidence boost. Go through the practice tests until you feel comfortable, and then you can go into the test knowing that you're ready for it.

Test Tips

On test day, you should be confident, knowing that you've prepared well and are ready to answer the questions. But aside from preparation, there are several test day strategies you can employ to maximize your performance.

First, as stated before, get a good night's sleep the night before the test (and for several nights before that, if possible). Go into the test with a fresh, alert mind rather than staying up late to study.

Try not to change too much about your normal routine on the day of the test. It's important to eat a nutritious breakfast, but if you normally don't eat breakfast at all, consider eating just a protein bar. If you're a coffee drinker, go ahead and have your normal coffee. Just make sure you time it so that the caffeine doesn't wear off right in the middle of your test. Avoid sugary beverages, and drink enough water to stay hydrated but not so much that you need a restroom break 10 minutes into the test. If your test isn't first thing in the morning, consider going for a walk or doing a light workout before the test to get your blood flowing.

Allow yourself enough time to get ready, and leave for the test with plenty of time to spare so you won't have the anxiety of scrambling to arrive in time. Another reason to be early is to select a good seat. It's helpful to sit away from doors and windows, which can be distracting. Find a good seat, get out your supplies, and settle your mind before the test begins.

When the test begins, start by going over the instructions carefully, even if you already know what to expect. Make sure you avoid any careless mistakes by following the directions.

Then begin working through the questions, pacing yourself as you've practiced. If you're not sure on an answer, don't spend too much time on it, and don't let it shake your confidence. Either skip it and come back later, or eliminate as many wrong answers as possible and guess among the remaining ones. Don't dwell on these questions as you continue—put them out of your mind and focus on what lies ahead.

Be sure to read all of the answer choices, even if you're sure the first one is the right answer. Sometimes you'll find a better one if you keep reading. But don't second-guess yourself if you do immediately know the answer. Your gut instinct is usually right. Don't let test anxiety rob you of the information you know.

If you have time at the end of the test (and if the test format allows), go back and review your answers. Be cautious about changing any, since your first instinct tends to be correct, but make sure you didn't misread any of the questions or accidentally mark the wrong answer choice. Look over any you skipped and make an educated guess.

At the end, leave the test feeling confident. You've done your best, so don't waste time worrying about your performance or wishing you could change anything. Instead, celebrate the successful completion of this test. And finally, use this test to learn how to deal with anxiety even better next time.

Review Video: <u>5 Tips to Beat Test Anxiety</u>
Visit mometrix.com/academy and enter code: 570656

Important Qualification

Not all anxiety is created equal. If your test anxiety is causing major issues in your life beyond the classroom or testing center, or if you are experiencing troubling physical symptoms related to your anxiety, it may be a sign of a serious physiological or psychological condition. If this sounds like your situation, we strongly encourage you to seek professional help.

Thank You

We at Mometrix would like to extend our heartfelt thanks to you, our friend and patron, for allowing us to play a part in your journey. It is a privilege to serve people from all walks of life who are unified in their commitment to building the best future they can for themselves.

The preparation you devote to these important testing milestones may be the most valuable educational opportunity you have for making a real difference in your life. We encourage you to put your heart into it—that feeling of succeeding, overcoming, and yes, conquering will be well worth the hours you've invested.

We want to hear your story, your struggles and your successes, and if you see any opportunities for us to improve our materials so we can help others even more effectively in the future, please share that with us as well. **The team at Mometrix would be absolutely thrilled to hear from you!** So please, send us an email (support@mometrix.com) and let's stay in touch.

If you'd like some additional help, check out these other resources we offer for your exam:

http://MometrixFlashcards.com/EMT

Additional Bonus Material

Due to our efforts to try to keep this book to a manageable length, we've created a link that will give you access to all of your additional bonus material.

Please visit https://www.mometrix.com/bonus948/emt to access the information.

GUARANTEED TO IMPROVE YOUR SCORE
"Effective, Affordable, Guaranteed"

At Mometrix, we think differently about tests. We believe you can perform better on your exam by implementing a few critical strategies and focusing your study time on what's most important. With so many demands on your time, you probably don't have months to spend preparing for an exam that holds the key to your future. Our team of testing experts devote hours upon hours to painstakingly review piles of content and boil it all down to the critical concepts that are most likely to be on your exam. **We do a lot of work cutting through the fluff to give you what you need the most to perform well on the exam.** But you don't have to take our word for it; here is what some of our customers have to say:

> *"I've just retaken my test and I scored way better than my previous score. I had this program for only 3 days and I just want to say that I can't believe how well it worked." - Mandy C.*

> *"Just wanted to say thank you. Due to your product I was able to ace my exam with very little effort. Your tricks did the trick. Thanks again, and I would recommend this product to anyone." - Erich L.*

> *"Just dropping you a note to let you know that I am completely satisfied with the product. I had already taken the test once and landed in the 75th percentile of those taking it with me. I took the test a second time and used some of your tips and raised my score to the 97th percentile. Thanks for my much improved score." - Denise W.*

> *"I just wanted to tell you I had ordered your study guide, and I finally aced the test after taking it numerous times. I tried tutors and all sorts of study guides and nothing helped. Your guide did the job and got me the score I needed! Thank you!" - Nicholas R.*

We offer study materials for over 1000 different standardized exams, including:

College Entrance Exams	**Teacher Certification Exams**
Medical/Nursing Exams	**Insurance Exams**
Financial Exams	**Dental Exams**
Military Exams	**Graduate & Professional School Exams**

Made in the USA
Middletown, DE
25 November 2019